CU00829082

Public Health and Globalisation

Why a National Health Service
Is Morally Indefensible

Iain Brassington

SOCIETAS
essays in political
& cultural criticism

imprint-academic.com

Published in the UK by Societas
Imprint Academic, PO Box 200, Exeter EX5 5YX, UK

Published in the USA by Societas
Imprint Academic, Philosophy Documentation Center
PO Box 7147, Charlottesville, VA 22906-7147, USA

ISBN 9781845400798

A CIP catalogue record for this book is available from the
British Library and US Library of Congress

Contents

This book is based on a paper, "Globalisation and the Moral Indefensibility of the NHS", presented at *Medicine and the Body Politic*, the inaugural conference of the Centre for Applied Philosophy, Politics and Ethics, University of Brighton, on 21 September 2006, and has benefited from discussions and conversations with other participants.

Introduction

How secure is the moral foundation for the National Health Service? Not, I shall argue here, as secure as all that.

This is not the same as saying that there is no secure moral foundation for a *public* health service; moreover, there might be political reasons to treat such a system as *national* health service, and practical reasons to administer a public health service on a national basis. Among the political reasons for there to be a national health service, we might count an argument along the lines that it is important to have a healthy population from which, say, effective armed forces can be recruited. But this clearly political motive would not work in a world in which there was no threat of war and so need for a soldiery. Correlatively, a claim that it is right that the state should ensure the fitness of the soldiery does make an appeal to rightness, and so an apparent appeal to moral considerations – but these are moral considerations in the service of political considerations. Similar considerations could be ventured in respect of other walks of life.

Might there be considerations, though, that would generate a reason to set up a body such as the NHS in a world without such political imperatives? After all, not all political reasons stand up to moral scrutiny, and sometimes we expect moral reasons to generate political reasons. For example, we tend not to think that apartheid should have been abolished just because it was politically expedient: we would probably tend to think that there was an independent moral reason to do so. The NHS itself makes a tacit appeal to a moral considerations that are not reducible to political imperatives as providing its basis, as we shall see (and assess) in chapter 2. So, although political and ethical arguments have been closely associated since at least the time of Aristotle, they are separable. Not all moral imperatives have to be reducible to political imperatives, and some moral imperatives generate political ones.

In respect of the practical argument – that a public health service is better organised on a national level – we might point out that this is not a moral argument for a national health service, so much as an argument about how to administer a public health service: if no public health service were required, though, the practical argument would evaporate, and could a service be run more efficiently by adverting to some other level, then we would have no reason to think in national terms.

Even if, as we go along, it turns out that there is no reliable moral foundation for the NHS, it will not follow from this that it is *wrong* for there to be such a body. Although some people might want to argue along those lines — in chapter 2, I shall mention, in passing, a line of argument that could be spun out to imply that there is something morally suspect about a great deal of public spending — others might satisfy themselves with the idea that a body such as the NHS is, at best, only a *partial* response to a moral imperative, and that, for it to be defensible, it ought to do more. It is compatible with this latter position to say that there is something at least *acceptable*, and quite possibly something *right*, about there being at least a minimal publicly-funded health service that is free at the point of delivery.

The Minimal Public Health Service

A minimal public health service would describe the barest morally acceptable health service, less than which we ought not to provide. If there is no successful argument for this minimal service, then there will be none available for a more-than-minimal service, of course: henceforward, I shall concern myself with arguments relating only to a minimal service. A minimal health service is, on this account, one that aims to provide such healthcare as is necessary to provide a reasonably long life that is reasonably comfortable.

Already, of course, this presents a problem, because a word like "reasonably" is vague, and so what counts as a reasonably long life may well be a matter of dispute. Still, there probably are some rules of thumb upon which we can rely without having to get too precise. For example, most people would agree that, though it is bad for an 80-year-old to die, his death is compatible with having lived a reasonably long life: mourn his passing as we may, we do not have to think that anything has gone seriously amiss when he dies, just because it is not unusual for people in their eighties to die. By contrast, if someone's life ends in his teens or before, we would probably be more likely to admit that something *had* gone amiss and that he had not lived a reasonably long life. The 80-year-old, we might say, has enjoyed a fair innings that the teenager has not. Naturally, we might prefer that neither dies—but, if there existed a magic potion that could give five extra years of life to one person and one alone, we would probably have no difficulty identifying the teenager as having a stronger claim to it; if the 80-year-old insisted that the extra years should go to him, but was not able to show that (or why) he was a special case, we might think him unreasonable, *just because* he is already fairly advanced in years. If this is compelling, although we might not be able to construct a particularly detailed account of what is a reasonably long life, we might still be able to make meaningful statements on the matter.

Similarly, though what counts as reasonable comfort is disputable, we can say that someone who thought that it involved never having a touch of eczema is probably mistaken, because such things are fairly minor irritants that might well be built into human life. Thus we might reasonably require that people simply learn to tolerate a little itching, especially if we are in a situation in which we have to decide whether to spend public money on them or on, say, treatments for diphtheria. We can say what it would be reasonable to use the resources on—and this means, again, that it is possible to make meaningful statements about a reasonable quality of life without having to be able to offer a precise definition of what this might amount to in reality.

Note that in all these attempt to get to grips with what is reasonable involve comparing one case with another. This is appropriate. For "reasonability" comes from the same root as "rationality", and ratiocination implies being able to strike a balance between two claims—to reach a ratio (and a ration). What it is reasonable to give to someone will depend, in part, on the context in which we are working. (This will be an important consideration in chapter 4.) Thus we might think it unreasonable to deny the magic potion to the 80-year-old if there was no competition for it, and unreasonable to deny the emollient to someone with eczema if she was the only person whom we could help. On the other hand, if we lived in such an implausibly rosy world, it might be unreasonable to expect us to contribute to a public health service at all. Is there really any great moral pressure for me to pay tax to provide magic potions so that 80-year-olds can live to 85? Would that be a reasonable demand to make?

Maybe it would; maybe not. I am not too concerned to answer the question here. For the time being, I will rest content with the idea that there is a moral case to be made in favour of there being at least a minimal publicly funded health service, which would aim to prevent deaths that we can agree are unreasonably early, and to prevent suffering that we can agree is unreasonably burdensome. On the face of it, this line of thought seems to give us the moral push necessary to give us something like the NHS.

However, my claim is that, once we have the moral momentum for a publicly funded body like the NHS, we cannot stop moving: we have seriously to contemplate some kind of *trans*national health service. This is why I think that there is no adequate moral defence for the NHS. If we think that a public health service is morally warranted, we cannot slam on the brakes and come to a halt as soon as we reach the nearest border post. We ought to think bigger.

Not to reach this conclusion would not really indicate an *error* in our moral thinking; it would, rather, indicate that our moral thought was incomplete. Arguments for an NHS are indefensible in the sense that there is no reason to think that the "National" part is warranted. In arguing for an NHS, one would not be arguing for something that is morally wrong; one would simply have failed to follow one's argument through to its proper conclusions. (In the same way, a student who admitted that the sum of the internal angles of a triangle is 180°, and that the sum of the two known internal angles is 120°, but who failed to deduce that the remaining unknown angle was 60°, would not have gone *wrong*: in a sense, he would not have gone *at all*. Generally, we would say that his failure to make the deduction was indefensible, in the sense that there is no adequate reason to explain it.) If we think that there should be public provision of healthcare, we ought to argue that the scope of that provision can, and should, be decoupled from national boundaries.

I shall claim in chapter 2 that this sort of consideration is particularly pertinent if we think that healthcare is something to which we can claim an entitlement. As we shall see, there is a good number of people who claim that healthcare is a right, and that it is a fundamental human right at that. If they are correct then we have a very good reason to suppose that anyone who counts as a human therefore has that right. It is not necessarily true to say that, because someone has a human right to something, it will fall to someone else to provide it — a separate argument would be necessary to make that step. But if that separate argument was to be made and we decided that we do have a moral reason to provide one person with something (such as healthcare) to which he has a right *just because* he is a human, then the same would seem to apply to all humans.

At the same time, if we think that the possession of a fundamental right to healthcare can be attributed to all humans, but deny that we thereby have a reason to *provide* it to any particular human, it would become difficult to see how *anyone* could claim that we owe it to them to provide that healthcare (although they might be able to make another claim to it based on their position as a holder of non-fundamental civil or political rights).

Put simply, if we think that no person is more or less human than any other, and if we think that healthcare is a human right, all humans presumably have an equal right to it. And if that right in one person is sufficient to generate an action from us of some sort, it ought to be the case that the same right in another person will be motivating as well. Moreover, because human rights make no reference to the nationality of the rights-holder, the nationality of Smith or Jones makes no difference to the question of whether we ought to supply healthcare to them as a matter of right. We have gone crashing through what is implied by an organisation such as a *national* health service.

Such a line might lead us to suppose that there ought to be equal amounts spent on healthcare on behalf of everyone in the world. I shall not argue here that all public health spending should be put into a global pot to be divided equally between the people of the world. A part of what I shall argue in the coming chapters is that it may well be permissible to treat some people differently from the way that one treats others, even if they can claim the same moral characteristics. Partiality is not a sin, and we do not have to treat everyone in the world alike. This is not a licence for all discrimination — some discrimination is clearly morally suspect, after all — but it does recognise that moral decision-making is not made from a God's-eye position.

Indeed, even if we have a duty to provide people with healthcare — and I shall outline in chapter 3 how we might want to argue along those lines — there is no particular reason to suppose that it is a duty that we owe to everyone in the same way. All the same, this will not make a national health service any less problematic. For the way that we divide up our duties need have nothing at all to do with nationality. Indeed, it would, I shall claim, be odd if they had anything more than a tangential relationship with questions of nationality. If we have duties to provide healthcare to others, or to contribute to a public health system, there is a good corresponding moral reason to avoid cramming it within national boundaries.

Notwithstanding this, I shall claim in chapter 4 that there *is* a strong moral case for *more* money to be sent overseas for the sake of healthcare there, and that if this means a greater sacrifice for us in the developed world in terms of the tax burden, or if it means cutting some services to which we have become used, then so be it. For even if we think that there is something special about the relationship between people within a nation that contributes towards a moral defence of a national health service – a claim that I shall deny but do not intend to try to refute – and that this contributes to an argument for the NHS's being, in the end, defensible, the fact that we spend so much on our own healthcare and so little on providing the means for people in the developing world to have access to healthcare should be something that we find troubling, provided that we accept a couple of moral claims that I think are pretty uncontroversial.

Setting the Scene

How much do we spend on the NHS, and how much does it cost us? The statistics that follow are all taken from data supplied by the World Bank's *World Development Indicators 2006*; and while some of the data refer to 2003 and others to 2004, they are sufficient to provide a picture – admittedly impressionistic – of some aspects of the world. According to the Bank's figures, per capita health spending in the UK in 2003 was $2428. This is equivalent to about 7.21% of per capita gross national income (GNI), which, in that year, stood at some $33 630. The vast majority of this health spending – 85.7% of the total – was concentrated in the public sector.

In the UK, the money that we spend on health buys us about a 78.5 year life expectancy: that is the average age that a person born today can hope to attain. Mortality among children under five years old runs at a rate of about 0.6%.

These figures compare very well with other parts of the world. Let's take for granted that sub-Saharan Africa is the poorest region in the world. In 2003, it had a population of 726 million, with a per capita GNI of $601. (Naturally, some individual countries are poorer: Ethiopia's population of 70 million got by on an average of $110 each per year). Within the sub-Saharan region, annual per capita expenditure on health was about $36 – just shy of 6% of GNI. In return for their spending, people living in the region can expect an under-5 mortality rate of around 17%; of those that survive, the life expectancy at birth for those born in 2004 was around 46.2 years (which is even worse than it was in 1990, by the way: we ought not to take even slow but steady improvements for granted).

We ought not to read too much into these raw statistics, of course. For those who care about statistical purity, jumping between 2003 and 2004 is likely to be an irritant. In my defence, I would point out that the difference between the two years is not likely to be all that great, and, at least for the sake of the broad argument I shall present here, it is not one that has to bother me. Another caveat is that the difference between the lower life expectancy in sub-Saharan Africa is not attributable solely to the fact that spending on health is so low: war, for example, accounts for a great number of premature deaths in the region, and for very few in the UK. People die younger in war zones. Still, even taking that into account, the picture in Africa is pretty grim: Swaziland, for example, is politically stable but has a life expectancy at birth of 57 and an under-5 mortality rate of 15.6%.

Another point that we might take into account is that a dollar simply buys more in some parts of the world than in others. And so we might think that simply saying who spends what on what is unreliable — we are not really comparing like with like. To correct for this latter kind of distortion, we can adjust average income by purchasing power parity (PPP). PPP is a way of comparing how far a dollar goes in various economies. Taking this into account, the PPP per capita GNI in sub-Saharan Africa is about $1842. Very roughly, this means that, if you took the $601 dollars that the average person earns in sub-Saharan Africa to the region and spent it all, the same shopping basket would cost $1842 in a hypothetical world market. More roughly still, $1 goes three times further in Africa than in the world economy as a whole. By contrast, the thirty-three and a half thousand dollars that the average citizen of the UK earns generates a per capita GNI adjusted for purchasing power of $31 430. Translated to health spending, the $36 dollars spent by each person in sub-Saharan Africa represent $110.16 of purchasing power at world prices, while the $2428 spent in the UK represent $2258 at world prices. This does close the gap a little — but not all that much.

It is not a problem that some people spend more on health than do others: people have different concerns. (For the sake of contrast, Americans spent $5711 each on health, equivalent to 13.8% of GNI and worth $5488 after adjusting for purchasing power: that is, about twice as much as the British measured as a proportion of GNI). And, anyway, sub-Saharan spending on health is, in relation to per capita GNI, in the ballpark of UK spending. Nor is it a problem that some people earn more than others: the fact that one is relatively poor does not mean that one is poor in absolute terms. Having said this, there is something startling about an income disparity that means that those in the UK enjoy an income 56 times higher than the average sub-Saharan with a purchasing power 17 times higher—and, of course, we know simply from watching the news that many people in the region are not just poorer than us, but that they are poor, *period*. It would be absurd to deny this.

Whatever we think of this sort of point, much of the argument that I present in the coming pages will be motivated by the observation that expenditure on health in the UK per capita in 2004 was over 4 times more than was earned *in total* by the average person living in sub-Saharan Africa. Were it possible to buy healthcare by the kilo, and taking into account PPP, we in the UK would have been able to buy over 20 kilos of it for every one bought in sub-Saharan Africa.

Given these statistics, I want to suggest that the moral arguments in favour of there being a body like the NHS should make this spending gap pretty well indefensible: even if my argument for thinking transnationally in respect of healthcare provision fails (and so the NHS *per se* is not, after all, indefensible), I think that there is still a strong case for thinking that the amount that we in the UK spend on healthcare for ourselves compared to that which we spend on the poorest in the world might very well be problematic. Either way, there is a case for much higher levels of transnational health spending.

Chapter 1

Public Health and Self-Interest

What would it take to convince a reasonable person that there ought to be a public health service? As I see it, there are three strategies that one might adopt, although there will be overlaps, and the degree of success we can expect from each is variable. The three strategies are based on an appeal to rights and a putative right to healthcare, which will be the focus of the next chapter; an appeal to duties that we have to provide for others' welfare, which will provide the focus of chapter 3; and appeals to self interest, which will provide my focus here.

Appeals to self interest, though they do provide *an* argument for a publicly-funded health service, do not provide all that *strong* an argument, and there is some truth in the notion that I want to get the weak argument out of the way first. However, to the extent that appeals to self interest do provide *some sort* of argument for a publicly-funded health service, they do not provide an argument for a *national* health service. In a pattern that we shall see repeated across the next two chapters, the arguments for publicly-funded healthcare turn out to be either arguments in favour of a parochial health service, or of a transnational health service.

Self Interest and Morality

Despite the intuitive feeling that many people have that self interest and moral demands are mutually antagonistic, there is no reason to suppose that this must be the case. We do not have to think that there is a conflict between acting in accordance with what is in our own interests and acting in a way that is demanded by commonsense morality. One reason for this is that it will turn out to be in our interests to act in accordance with commonsense moral rules. Very roughly, the idea here might be something along the lines that our lives will be made easier if we act in what most people would accept as a reasonably decent sort of a way, if only because a sustained failure to act in a reasonably decent sort of a way will increase the possibility of our being lynched by angry neighbours. Membership of society confers on us certain benefits such as security, and so we have an incentive to tailor our behaviour to fit society's expectations. This might mean that, on occasion, we have to sacrifice certain short-term opportunities; still, the longer-term benefits of such self-control will make the sacrifice worth it.

The problem with this account is that it does not really get rid of selfish actions, and the idea that I should accommodate social norms into my behaviour is only really compelling if I am scared that I will not get away with acting on my most immediate desire. If I am an accomplished thief, I will not have to worry about falling foul of the norm against theft. Moreover, such an account does not tell us how those social norms appeared in the first place, or even anything much about their content. It is all very well to say that there is no necessary conflict between self-interest and obedience to moral norms, but it there might still be a dispute about what those norms are and how they arrived on the scene.

Such a worry can be avoided by adverting to another account of self interest that takes its lead from the thought of Thomas Hobbes (1588–1679), and it is by following a Hobbesian line that we come across another reason to suppose that there is no conflict between commonsense morality and self interest. In *Leviathan*, Hobbes' most famous work, he argues for the claim that the system of behavioural laws that we lump together under the word "morality" is an expression of certain basic laws of nature. Among these laws is that each organism is concerned for its own survival and wellbeing. In other words, commonsense morality grows from self interest. Hobbes' argument is detailed, but it can be paraphrased.

The argument begins with the denial that there is anything absolutely good or evil: moral epithets, Hobbes thinks, simply reflect our desire or contempt for something. Now, absent any set of rules to govern our behaviour, we would find ourselves in a "state of nature". Such a state would represent a "Warre; and such a warre, as is of every man, against every man" as each of us tries to establish his own security and welfare. The cumulative effect of this war is that

> [i]n such condition, there is no place for Industry; because the fruit thereof is uncertain: and consequently no Culture of the Earth; no Navigation, nor use of the commodities that may be

> imported by Sea; no commodious Building; no Instruments of
> moving, and removing such things as require much force; no
> Knowledge of the face of the Earth; no account of Time; no Arts;
> no Letters; no Society; and which is worst of all, continuall feare,
> and danger of violent death; And the life of man, solitary, poore,
> nasty, brutish, and short. (Hobbes, 1996, p 89)

Such a situation would clearly be undesirable; however, humans have the insight to realise that, by concerted action and the institution of laws that limit conduct, it is possible to emerge from a state of nature and to have a more desirable life. Through negotiation, we will end up with a system of rules that will protect each of us from each other, and because the safety that we obtain in that way is both desirable in its own terms and conducive to more desirable things, we will have an incentive to adopt that system.

Hobbes' intention is to provide an account for how a State grows out of human rationality, and how it is rational for us to prefer any Sovereign over a state of nature—but what is important for my purposes is simply the idea that a system of rules that govern how we behave can arise out of self interest. So we have an incentive to agree rules of behaviour; and, on the basis that anyone who discovers we are bending or breaking the rules is likely to make life difficult for us, we have an incentive to adopt them and stick to them as well. But "rules of behaviour" is simply a way of talking about morality—bear in mind the earlier denial that there is anything simply and absolutely good or evil. Thus there is not a conflict or tension between morality and self interest: the opposite is the case. Morality is the *expression* of self-interest among rational and cooperative agents.

Because I am not interested in Hobbes *per se*, I can leave the exposition of his thought at that. What counts here is that we can generate a list of things that we ought to do from a sufficiently careful analysis of what we want to achieve for ourselves and the ways in which we might go about getting them. Indeed, even if the idea that morality emerges from self interest turns out to be erroneous there is clearly still a number of times when an action carried out specifically for self interested reasons is compatible with what commonsense morality might well demand. For example, a shopkeeper's decision not to short-change his customer might be attributable to the belief that that would be the wrong thing to do, but it might be attributable to the belief that the best way to keep customers is not to short-change them: in other words, the same action might arise equally easily from simple pragmatism as from more traditional "moral" considerations (which turn out to be based on pragmatism anyway).

The Self Interest-Based Argument for Public Healthcare

If we think that there ought to be something like a publicly-funded health service, it is possible that this "ought" simply indicates what moral philosophers call a *hypothetical imperative*. A hypothetical imperative takes the form: if you want this, do that. If I want to be a better pianist, I ought to practise more, and I ought to practise more even though noone would say that I would be any less of a decent person for not practising (since many decent people are awful pianists). Granted that people are concerned to provide for their own welfare and are interested in living as long and as comfortable a life as possible — that is, they are motivated by self interest in at least some of what they do — it is at least possible that this could generate a hypothetical argument along the lines that they ought to support the foundation of a publicly-funded health service.

It might not be immediately clear how this jump is made, but the gap between acting out of a concern for one's own welfare and providing a public health service is one that we can navigate tolerably nimbly. Having said this, it is worth noting that the claim implicit in what comes over the rest of the chapter (and, with appropriate modifications, the rest of the book) is not so much that self interest *does* generate a reason to found a publicly funded health service as it is that *if* we think that self interest generates a reason to found a publicly funded health system, *then* we ought to think this and that about it. For this reason, although the arguments that I am about to present rely on many contingencies obtaining that may not obtain in the real world, the general validity of the considerations ought not to be affected.

The first step is simply to point out that we would be irrational not to provide for and to seek to maximise our welfare whenever possible. Of course, the real world is such that there will often be constraints on the ease with which we can do this; and there may even be situations in which we might think it wrong to be concerned primarily with our own welfare — for example, a parent who neglected her child because she was more concerned about herself might provoke strong moral censure. Nevertheless, all else being equal, we can take it as read that people can, do and may seek to make their own lives as good as possible whenever possible, and that a failure to do so might well indicate something psychologically puzzling about the person in question.

If this is correct — and there is not much chance of it not being — it means that a rational person has an incentive to make some sort of provision for his healthcare needs. An assessment of what he expects those needs to be will tell him how much provision he needs to make. At the outside, this might mean that someone who is confident that he will never need any healthcare will have no incentive to make any provision for it. However, ordinary mortals can be reasonably confident that they will, at some point, find themselves capable of benefiting from some kind of health intervention, and that providing for such an eventuality would be wise. Naturally, there is also a reason to ensure that the impact of the need for healthcare intervention is as low as possible, since it obviously does not serve anyone's interest to have to make more of a sacrifice than strictly necessary to ensure his welfare goals.

There are several ways in which we could seek to provide for our own future welfare. One method would be to stuff a certain amount of money under the mattress every week and thereby hope that we will have enough set aside to cover the cost of any operation that we may need in the future. Such a policy would serve as a primitive kind of insurance. The obvious downside is that anyone following such a policy may find that he falls ill next week, before having built up sufficient to pay for the treatment, or that he falls victim to a serious illness that he hadn't expected as a real possibility when he was deciding how much he needed to put aside and the cost of curing it is therefore beyond his reach. And, of course, someone following this strategy may never fall ill, but be killed outright many years hence by a bus. Such a person would have wasted his money.

A second method of ensuring that we could get hold of the healthcare that we will need would be to make a contribution to a private insurance fund. The benefits of private insurance over mattress-stuffing are several. In the first place, it ought not to matter if one falls ill the week after the first premium is paid — the company is gambling that you will not (more: it is gambling that you will live a long and healthy life before being killed outright by a bus, because that means their income will be maximised and their outgoings minimised), but it will be contractually bound to pay out if the gamble does not pay off. Therefore there should be no worry about not having built up enough of a stash to pay for treatment. Similarly, the company will be gambling that, even if it does have to pay out, it will not have to pay out *much*. But, again, if the necessary treatment is expensive, it will (assuming it is a well regulated insurer) cover it. Of course, the insurer's gamble might pay off: any one of us might live on and on, apparently indestructible, until that encounter with a bus. In that case, the premiums paid would have been, in a sense, wasted. But, as well as cover for healthcare interventions, a private insurance policy could also be taken as buying the confidence that our healthcare fund would be highly unlikely to be exhausted — and this confidence is worth having in its own right. Moreover, sustained good health might mean that our premiums would fall over time without adversely affecting the cover available to us. This point would not be true for the mattress-stuffers. Finally, an insurance scheme ought to generate economies of scale that make it more efficient than mattress-stuffing.

Finally, the healthcare that we need could also be provided by a publicly funded health service. The advantages of public funding over mattress-stuffing are comparable to those offered by a healthcare system funded by private contributions. There is, though, a disadvantage, in that, while a private insurer could choose not to cover certain people if they look as though they will be costly, a healthcare system that relied on public funding would find such a policy difficult to maintain, and so the costly would have to be covered, possibly to the detriment of others. A private insurer is a shopkeeper of a certain sort with goods to sell, and, to this extent, he can choose to whom he is going to sell his goods. Just as a casino owner might refuse entry to someone who has a reputation for counting cards because, even if we choose to describe card-counting as exploiting a skill rather than cheating, such a customer would prove costly, so an insurer might choose not to sell a policy to a customer who is likely to prove costly to him. By contrast, while a publicly-funded system might encourage people to alter their lifestyle, and might legitimately refuse *some* non-basic treatments to people who refused to do so, it could not really refuse to treat them *wholesale*. Therefore the premiums paid into a public health system might, if the contingencies work out right, be slightly larger than those that we might expect to pay in a private system in order to cover these eventualities.

On the other hand, just because everyone is covered by a public system, we might find that the premiums are much more widely spread, and, just because they are paid by everyone (including those who will claim little in return), the difference might be minimal. On top of this, several commentators have pointed out that some people might contribute disproportionately to public health funds: smokers, for example, pay a large amount in tax, but, just because they tend to die young by comparison to non-smokers, do not suffer from the diseases of old age so much and so do not represent such a drain on the health service as we might expect (see Wilkinson, 1999, for a useful roundup of arguments along these lines). This being the case, we might be in a position to suppose that insurance premiums might be kept low, paradoxically enough, by the inclusion of high-risk groups in a public insurance scheme.

All this said, though, there is not (I will admit) all that much difference between the version of self interest that provides an incentive for private health insurance and that which seeks to generate a publicly-funded system of healthcare provision, and I shall treat them as being so far, to all intents and purposes, equally attractive to the aggregate of rational self interested agents. Still, the considerations so far have taken it as read that agents live more or less in isolation from each other. And, as we know, that is not what happens in reality.

It is clear that our own welfare is tied up with the welfare of those around us, and it is not difficult to point to any number of everyday examples that establish this point. If a colleague or the person sitting next to me on the train has a cold and that cold is contagious, then there is a chance that I will get it too. There is not a great deal that can be done about that. So a concern to maximise my own welfare will mean, in practice, either that at least some account has to be taken of the welfare of those around me so that they do not indirectly threaten to diminish my welfare, or that I ought to attempt to minimise the effect that others will have on my welfare without much regard for theirs.

This second option might represent quite a tall order. One way that I might think that I could minimise the risk to my welfare presented by others would be to avoid human contact altogether, but this is a non-starter, for there is reason to think that humans are social by nature, and need other humans to flourish — Aristotle articulates this point eloquently at the start of his *Politics* (Aristotle, 1992, esp. 1253a1ff and 1253a29ff). If I cut myself off from humanity completely, I might well find that I am reducing, rather than guaranteeing, my welfare: as well as diminishing the risks arising from human contact, I will also have limited my access to the benefits. The life of the germ-free hermit is sterile in more than one sense.

Pursuing some other means of ensuring that others present little risk to my welfare without having to deal directly with their health status is likely to prove impractical. At its least impractical, it would mean that I should be willing to consider wearing a surgical mask while on the train to minimise the risks from contagious fellow-passengers. Such a strategy is onerous, and is far from foolproof anyway.

If we are self interested, it might occur to us, too, that it is better for there not to be a risk than to have to manage it. This kind of thought would, if I was motivated solely by a concern for my interests, give me a reason to support moves that would increase the general level of health in the population at large. Note that I would not have to care about anyone else's welfare in its own terms: I would simply have to be aware that providing some minimal guarantee of others' welfare would be a way (quite possibly a way among others) for me to guarantee my own welfare. In other words, a self interested position does seem capable of generating an argument for public healthcare in at least a minimal sense. And such healthcare would bring with it a virtuous circularity, as well: for the higher a person's general level of health, the better will he be able to deal with any new risks to his health that come along. By extension, the healthier the population at large, the better able it will be to cope with contagion. Health creates health, and so the burden of providing that health might be something that we could expect to diminish over time.

(Of course, I would also have an interest to ensure that the burden of funding this health service was carried by others — but, on the basis that I also have an interest in not antagonising the rest of society, wisdom might suggest making a contribution of my own.)

Health and Wealth

If self interest is our main motivator, other considerations could be brought to the table as well that would bolster the argument for at least a minimal public health service. For one thing, it is not only my health that is tied up with other people's; my wealth is, too.

In the quotation from Hobbes that I used a while ago, we can see the claim that one of the characteristics of the life of man in the state of nature is that it is "poore". When we are force to live in a situation that can be described as a war of all against all, there is no place for industry or the commodious products of industry: the fruits of industry are uncertain, and, in such a war, people have better things to do anyway, such as ensuring basic survival. Cooperation makes our lives better, Hobbes thinks. Similar considerations might apply to health provision. In a world in which people are forced to fend for themselves in respect of healthcare, we would expect the general standard of health to be lower. But a lower general standard of health will mean that people are less productive: industry and the commodious products of industry will suffer.

More generally, the economy is less buoyant the less healthy people are: the Confederation of British Industry estimates that sick leave cost the UK economy £13 billion in 2005, with 164 million working days lost. Even allowing for absenteeism (which the CBI allows occurs at a rate of about 13%), this represents a large loss to the economy.

This loss impacts on each of us. The more buoyant an economy, the higher the general levels of wealth in that economy. It is therefore rational for a self interested person to want the economy to perform as well as possible; even someone who does not benefit directly from a buoyant economy is likely to benefit indirectly, and everyone is more *likely* to be wealthier in a buoyant economy than in a stagnant one. Now, if one of the ways in which we can maximise the buoyancy of an economy is to ensure that its participants are as healthy as possible — as seems to be the case — then it would seem to follow that a self interested person has an interest in the other participants in the economy in which he participates being as healthy as possible. Rational self interest, moreover, might turn out to demand that some contribution is made to the general welfare as a result: even if we would be better off if everyone had insurance that covered just their own welfare, not everyone *does* have such cover, and their inability to provide for themselves as high a level of welfare as possible could well turn out to be detrimental to our ability to provide for ourselves to the extent that we might wish. For as long as any contribution that he makes to a public health system will pay for itself in the long term (in financial terms as well as simply not antagonising the neighbours), it is something that a rational self interested person ought to embrace.

This amounts to the claim that rational self interest provides an incentive to support at least the principle of a publicly funded health system that can guarantee at least minimal healthcare provision for all, irrespective of whether they have private health cover. Whether or not one supports the practical application of this principle might be another matter — it might be that no contribution will, in the real world, pay for itself; and, even if it would, a self interested person will always have an incentive to minimise his own contribution, possibly to the extent of ducking out of any contribution at all, when the marginal impact of such minimisation is low. However, I shall concentrate on the principle.

The point that, if the contingencies work out aright, it may be in the interests of a rational and self interested agent to contribute towards providing healthcare for members of the public at large. Economies of scale and the sheer impracticality of contributing to a private health cover scheme proportionally to the impact that this or that other person has on one's own welfare mean that a public health scheme is, by far, a better option than private cover (though, of course, none of this militates against a person's right to continue to contribute to any private scheme that he wants). Moreover, there is the strong possibility of another virtuous circle emerging under such a system: the healthier the population, the wealthier; the wealthier people are, the more they will be able to contribute to public and/ or private health provision, and so the higher the general level of health. This increased health means fewer days off work and more wealth creation, and so on.

The picture I have just provided is not intended to serve as an argument for a public health service. Rather, the point is to show how, if we think that self interest is or ought to be the primary factor that motivates people, such a factor could, if the circumstances are right, translate to an argument for a publicly funded health service. The argument would be supportable; whether or not the premises obtain, reliant as they are on empirical claims about the way that the economic considerations stack up, is not really my concern here. Indeed, even if a self interest-based argument was forthcoming, just because it would rely for its normative punch on real-world conditions that may or may not obtain, it would be very weak.

But still, the conclusion of even a weak argument, and the implications of such an argument, can be interesting. If we are convinced by any incipient argument for a public health service, one of the interesting implications is that it would not be a *national* health service. The self interest-based arguments for a *public* health service are, in fact, arguments for a *trans*national health service.

Self Interest and Transnationalism

The underlying thought here is that there is no reason to suppose that those to whose welfare my own welfare is related need be my compatriots; and, if my welfare is related to my compatriots' welfare, this need not be the whole story.

If we look at the considerations that would seem to serve as incentives for the provision of a public health service, we will see without too much difficulty why a putative public health service ought to be transnational. In the first place, if our concern is to ensure that we are as free from contagion as possible, then it takes very little to point out that our concern is not limited by, and has little to do with, national boundaries. This is a point that, in its own terms, is so trivial as to be hardly worth making. However, inasmuch as our concern for our own welfare gives us an indirect reason to take some concern in others' welfare, there is consequently no reason why this concern should be limited to national boundaries. Indeed, depending on how we look at things, it might give a reason to *resist* any such body as a national health service on one of three grounds: first, that it would be too demanding; second, that it would not be comprehensive enough; and third, a combination of the two.

The idea that a national health service might be too demanding arises from the realisation that the people who present the highest risk of contagion to a person are those whom he sees every day, and such is the nature of most people's lives that they will be not only his compatriots, but also people who live in a fairly limited geographical area: people living in Cornwall and people living in Kirkwall rarely cross paths. Indeed, people living only a short walk from each other may rarely cross paths. If this is correct, it will present the self interested agent with a motive to contribute to a fairly small-scale health service, but not a great deal else—something on the scale of a nation (especially when that nation is the size of the UK) would be unwarranted. After all, just because people whom one encounters only seldom present little danger to one's own welfare, one would not benefit from providing healthcare resources for them. Therefore considerations based on self interest would not only fail to counsel in favour of making such a move, but would counsel more positively against it.

So this would give us one reason to think that a national health service was unwarranted. On the other hand, other considerations might lead us to suppose that the service that we *do* have an incentive to support would have a scope that would not be bounded by the same limits within which a notional national health service would have to work. For one thing, though I might not cross paths with people who live more than a short walk from me all that often, it might well be the case that I do cross paths with at least some people who live a good distance from me—in other countries, in fact. (I shall not comment on the fact that, in some places, one's nearest neighbour might live in a different country—and I am even told that there is a restaurant on the Slovenia-Croatia border where the till is in one country and the toilets in another — though the possibility of such a situation is obviously relevant here.) If it is concern to protect myself and my interests that leads me to contribute to others' welfare, it would plainly be something less than rational for me to suppose that nationality is all that important here. I can just as easily contract an illness from a foreigner as from a compatriot. In a world in which I travel, some foreigners' health might well be more of a concern to me than most of my compatriots'.

This point is compounded by the obvious fact that the people we meet frequently also meet other people just as frequently. Hence, although we might rightly feel that those people who are only on the periphery of our social circle (or not in it at all) represent *less* of a risk to us than others, they will not for all that present no risk at all. Given that the world in which we live is enormously interconnected, it would perhaps be foolhardy to suppose that *anyone* presents a negligible risk, even though that risk might be indirect. (The idea that there are only six degrees of separation between any two living people on the face of the planet might be roped in here as a nice illustration of the point.) Very brutally, if some aspect of our welfare depends on another's wellbeing, and if his wellbeing is related to that of a third person, then we cannot really say that that third person has nothing to do with us. We need not be as concerned about his welfare as about that of the person close to us, and certainly not as much as about our own: still, we cannot discount him entirely. Fully-informed rational self interest means that we have at least to consider providing minimal healthcare facilities for people of whom we are, at most, dimly aware.

The mere fact that the world is commonly thought of as much smaller today than it has been at any time in the past means that a reasonable self interested person cannot act as though what is going on close to him represents all about which he needs to concern himself. Because I, and people I know, insist on travelling abroad, sometimes to benighted parts of the world and sometimes simply to places where other forms of disease are endemic, the fact is that there is no reliable way of saying that some medical problems in one part of the world will not become medical problems in another.

The example of the SARS virus in 2003 and persistent worries about the H5N1 strain of influenza provide good illustrations of this point, for they are instances in which a health problem that, only a couple of generations ago, might have been serious in one part of the world but not have presented any cause for worry to those living on the other side, appear to have become a threat to everyone in the world. The first reported SARS fatality was in Vietnam—but the condition was also reported in Canada within weeks. It would not have taken all that much for SARS to be a much bigger problem than it turned out to be—a small difference caused by a random mutation in its genome, perhaps, might have meant that it became much more deadly. As it was, the disease apparently came from out of nowhere but labs were able to deal with it reasonably quickly. But it could easily have come out of nowhere and presented a much greater problem. This is not meant to provide a point about self interest *per se*—however, the point is that *if* self interest means that we have a reason to be concerned about the health of others around us (as seems to be a fair supposition), the scope of this care is, in principle, indefinite.

The fact that SARS did present a problem and could have presented a bigger one might be taken as evidence that, regardless of the interest that rational self interested people might take in providing healthcare in other parts of the world, some diseases will simply appear from time to time about which we will be able to do very little. This is almost certainly true. However, the risk of impotence does not generate an argument for inaction, and the point remains that a population that is generally healthy is less vulnerable to new diseases than one that is not. Healthy people are more likely to be able to fight off a disease quickly, and so present less of a risk to others. In the event that a disease kills someone, those charged with disposing of the body will be less endangered themselves if they are generally healthy and not having to deal with other infections as they do their work.

Of course, one response of this kind of point might be simply to place more restrictions on travel and international trade: if internationalism means that we are at risk from disease from around the world, then self interest would seem to give us a reason to restrict that internationalism. This is true—but the reasons that we have to restrict internationalism might well be countered by other reasons not to. We would almost certainly lose out from such a move, and it is not clear in any way that its benefits would warrant the costs.

We could, additionally, insist that anyone who travels abroad is well provided with vaccinations, mosquito repellent and so on to minimise the risk that they will inadvertently serve as a vector for contagious disease. But such a system would be unworkable. Not only would it be massively cumbersome, but it would also fail to neutralise a significant part of the putative danger. After all, the people whose movements are the easiest to track are those who follow established routes, and those who follow established routes tend to be from the wealthier ends of the social spectrum, which means that they tend to be exactly those who enjoy the best health and can afford better healthcare in the first place. By contrast, those who are poorer and so more likely to act as disease vectors are more likely to be the people whose travel between countries is along informal routes – here, we might think about people who are smuggled into Europe in containers or on rubber dinghies from North Africa. But, just because their movements around the world are informal, it means that those who are the most likely to act as disease vectors are also the very people whose movements are least susceptible to regulation and in respect of whom it is the most difficult to enforce a vaccination policy. If a bacterium was looking for a way to travel to new parts of the world, it could do little better than to hitch a ride on an illegal immigrant. And this generates an incentive among the self interested to minimise the vulnerability to disease of the poorest.

Deciding only to vaccinate myself against possible diseases rather than providing health resources to others is not likely to be the best strategy if it is self interest that motivates me. For one thing, there is no effective vaccination against some disease, which means that a generally healthy population is still the best means of preventing infection. For another, self-vaccination will also not save me from the economic problems associated with other people getting ill. So there is no conceptual difficulty in accepting the claim that providing the means to improve the general level of health around the world is a better way for me to protect my interests, correctly identified, than simply vaccinating myself. Inescapably, I may very well be better off the healthier the world in which I reside. This implies a reasonably healthy general population not just on a local scale, but on the scale of everyone who is, or who could be, a participant in the world economy. And, just because of the interdependence of economies today, this means just about everyone. In other words, if we stand to benefit from international trade, then, *qua* rational self interested agents, we ought at least to consider the benefits of making some contribution to ensure a basic level of health in the populations with whom we could be trading.

Moreover, if there is the possibility that we might get into virtuous circles when it comes to ensuring that those around us are healthy, either because a healthy general population is less vulnerable to illness or because the world economy is more buoyant and more supportive of the trade that provides wealth when as many people as possible can participate in it, then there is no reason to suppose that they will be any less virtuous or any less circular when the arguments are made on a scale that takes no account of national boundaries.

A self interested agent has a reason to provide for the health of those around him, whether or not they are his compatriots. A public health service might well turn out to serve his interests. A health service that is *a priori* national will be less likely to do this. If this kind of argument fails to generate pressure for the provision of basic healthcare across national boundaries, it is only because of the way that the economic contingencies stack up; but such a reliance on economic contingencies also means that the argument is likely to fail to generate much in the way of pressure for the provision of basic healthcare *within* countries as well. In other words, irrespective of the weakness or strength of any incentive to provide any kind of public health service that can be ascribed to arguments based on appeals to self interest, the considerations operative are equally operative on a national and a transnational level. There is no reason to draw a distinction.

If we are drawn by self interest to demand a public health service but think that this implies a *national* health service, we have made a mistake. A mistaken conclusion is indefensible, almost as a matter of definition. We ought, if we have considered matters aright, to look transnationally.

Chapter 2

Public Health and Rights

Self interest provides only a weak motivation to establish a public health service. But to the extent that it provides any motivation at all, the service that it would establish would be transnational rather than national: to attempt either to limit its scope to within national boundaries or to extend it as *far* as national boundaries would indicate either that some factor beyond self interest had influenced our thought on the matter, or that our thought was simply inconsistent or incomplete. Whatever the explanation, a *national* health service cannot be presented as something warranted or demanded by following the directives of self interest. If it is narrow self interest that drives our actions, we will lack a reason to support anything as expansive as a national health service; if it is a wider self interest that drives us, we will regard national boundaries as mere scenery.

A much stronger case for a publicly funded health service can be presented if we appeal to the notion of rights, and the manner in which an appeal to rights might be used to provide the moral basis for a public health service is what I intend to look at in this chapter. This is not to say that any fully worked-out appeal to rights is straightforward. In the first place, we have to decide whether our ostensible right to this or that is a *human* right or a *civil* right. A human right, unsurprisingly, is something that we have courtesy of belonging to the correct species; and, because it is difficult to see how one could stop belonging to a species, it is something that is, to all intents and purposes, inalienable, enduring in each of us for as long as we are human. (That a human right is inalienable does not mean that an inalienable right is a human right, of course: we might think that all sentient beings have a right not to have suffering inflicted on them, and this would therefore apply inalienably to most—though probably not all—animals, as well as to humans.) Having said this, that a right is inalienable does not mean that it cannot be overridden. Free speech is something that many people take to be a human right, but this does not mean that there is no time at which others might legitimately tell us to shut up: classically, my right to speak freely does not mean that I have a right to gossip throughout the theatrical performance; nor does it mean that I have the right to be gratuitously offensive, since most points can be made in a more moderate tone. Free speech therefore simply means that, in those circumstances in which I have the opportunity to speak, the content of what I say is up to me, subject to considerations about incitement and so on. If we think that healthcare is a human right, by the same token, it might be something to which my right is inalienable, but which can be trumped on some occasions by other factors.

By contrast, our entitlement to some other things comes by dint of civil rights. There is a strong expectation that human rights get protected as civil rights — we tend to criticise governments that do not allow the exercise of what we hold to be human rights. But there are also things that we can claim as a right only because of our being a member of the right polity, which is to say that human rights do not provide the foundation for some civil rights. For example, in some parts of the world, one has the right to ride a motorcycle without a helmet; in others, there is no such right. And it would be hard to see how one had one's human rights violated by being forced to ride with a helmet, since it is perfectly possible to deny that there is any such right *to* violate in the first place.

It is easy enough to see how one might come by civil rights: all it takes is for the powers that be — whether power is held by an absolute monarch, enlightened despot or the *demos* as a whole is immaterial here — to say that the people, henceforward, have a right to do this or that. Nor is it difficult to see how we might identify what "this or that" indicates: in the majority of cases, there need be no great puzzle concerning whether or not we are entitled to something as a matter of civil right — all we have to do is find the relevant statute. It is more difficult, though, to see how we might come to be holders of human rights — even though we have become used to thinking that there is such a thing — and also more difficult to see how we can tell what it is to which we apparently have a human right.

Part of the problem here is identifying exactly how it is that membership of a particular species, or the possession of particular characteristics, generates a *right*. I shall not attempt to solve this problem here. Nonetheless, if we trace the evolution of rights-thinking, the idea that there might be such a thing as a natural right was beginning to crystallise by the seventeenth century — Brenda Almond notes the idea that the English political crises of the mid- and late-seventeenth century might mark the birth-pangs of the modern concept of a right (Almond, 1993). From a concept of natural rights, it is not difficult to see the genesis of a concept of human rights. An important aspect of the growth of a belief in natural or human rights is that it is not up to the state to grant them, but that it *is* up to the state to protect or accommodate them. This is a reversal of the state's role in respect of a civil right such as riding a motorcycle without a helmet, since no such right exists without the state's say-so and, if it does exist, it is liable to revocation by the state.

Some people are moved to deny that there is any such thing as a human right: Jeremy Bentham (1748–1832), for example, famously described the idea of an inalienable natural right as "nonsense upon stilts". For Bentham and those of a similar mind, because the moral value of an act or event is a function of its propensity to generate wel-fare, and because value has to be accounted for in empirical terms, welfare considerations not only have the ability to trump rights: there is simply no room in the picture for rights at all. At the outside, talk of rights might serve as an elegant fiction invoked as a means to achieve some welfare end — people might be on the whole better off if each of us acted *as if* there were such a thing as a right — but that does not mean that there *really* is any such thing as a right. And Bentham does not provide the only criticism of rights-thought: Marxists, for example, have it within their power to insist that appeals to "rights" only ever gloss social considerations. Thus we might, under Marxist or some similar critical tutelage, claim that a so-called human right is basically a property right that one has over oneself or one's body. But property rights are simple functions of economic relationships, not of anything deeper. If this kind of think-ing is attractive, we will not have denied the importance or existence of rights (*à la* Bentham) so much as debunked any appeal to them.

Nevertheless, let us allow that an appeal to a concept such as rights is not entirely *de trop*: that the idea of a right has a respectable place in moral argument, and that at least some rights are *human* rights, and therefore inalienable from anyone who is human or who possesses that characteristic that makes members of the species *homo sapiens* morally different from other species so far discovered. We might still wonder what would appear on a list of human rights: of particular import here would be the question of whether health or healthcare were things to which we could lay a claim as a matter of right.

The idea that we have a right of any sort to health or being healthy is a non-starter: although it would be terrifically *nice* if we could pass the duration of our lives without illness, one simply has no *right* to be healthy any more than one has a right to be wealthy or to win the lottery. It makes no sense at all to claim that a rhinovirus has violated any of our rights by causing us to have a cold. However, there is still room to ask whether health*care* might be something to which we can lay claim as a matter of right; whether, if it is, that right is civil in nature or more fundamental; and what is implied by the answers that we give to these questions.

The Right to Healthcare

The idea that people have anything like a fundamental or human right to healthcare could well be contentious. Yet, irrespective of whether there is in reality any such right, we can talk meaningfully about the scope of a hypothetical right just as easily as we can talk about the scope of a real one. Moreover, the fact that we can talk about the scope of a hypothetical right means that I do not have to spend too much time worrying about whether there is any such right, nor about whether it is a human right or simply civil. Instead, I shall simply concentrate on what we ought to think granted the supposition that talk of human rights is meaningful and that included on the list of human rights is a right to healthcare. It is this claim that will fuel the argument as it unfolds through the chapter.

It is worth noting that a putative human right to healthcare is taken seriously by many. Not least among them is the NHS itself, the website of which claims that healthcare is a basic human right. The NHS' claim, meanwhile, echoes that of Article 25 of the Universal Declaration of Human Rights, which states that

> [e]veryone has the right to a standard of living *adequate for the health and well-being of himself* and of his family, *including* [...] *medical care* and necessary social services, and the right to security in the event of unemployment, sickness, disability, widowhood, old age or other lack of livelihood in circumstances beyond his control. [Emphasis mine]

I shall take the UN, and, perhaps more importantly, the NHS, at their word and see where they take us.

In accordance with the points I made in chapter 1, I shall assume that any claims that we make about a right to healthcare are most likely to succeed if our ambitions are kept reasonably low — that is, that the scope of the right to healthcare is limited. Even if there is a right to healthcare, we do not have to think that there is for that reason a right to every conceivable healthcare intervention, especially given the restrictions of a finite planet. Hence, for example, we might suppose that there is a sustainable argument for there being a right to emergency treatment for a heart attack, but we need not suppose that there is a right to bypass surgery. In other contexts, there might be a right to decent care (including palliative care) if we get cancer, but no right to at least some cancer drugs. Even if we all agree that it would be very good if we could have every possible treatment, we do not have to agree that there is any *rights* claim to be made to that effect.

Of course, neither the NHS' claim nor the UN's directly leads to a claim that there ought to be national health service; in fact, they do not directly lead to a claim that there even ought to be a *public* health service. Nor, strictly speaking, does any claim about a right to healthcare imply that it is up to the state to provide it any more than the claim that one has a right to read books means that the state is obliged to provide them (although we would be entitled to expect the state to respect this right, take it seriously, and therefore refrain from banning them). It certainly does not follow from the claim that there is any right to receive healthcare that is free at the point of delivery. However, it takes little more than a sprightly hop, skip and jump from here to provide an argument that, at the very least, free basic healthcare ought to be provided by someone and that it ought to be the public sector, which would almost certainly be represented by the state, that provides it.

Let us imagine a world in which the right to healthcare is taken to mean no more than that noone has a right to act to prevent a person accessing healthcare; healthcare is available, but only from those private sector bodies that are willing to enter the market. (If it should happen that no private body is willing to provide healthcare, there would simply be none to be had beyond what one can provide for oneself.) In this world, the ill are presented with a bill for every intervention; naturally, there is no reason why it might not be possible to buy insurance to cover these bills. So healthcare is provided on much the same basis as any other good or service. It might be suggested that the role of the state in such a setup is, at most, to ensure that the healthcare market is reasonably well regulated. (Why it should fall to the state to ensure that the market was well-regulated is something with which I shall deal, albeit glancingly, in a little while.) Because healthcare is just like any good or service, the same rules about paying for it obtain as obtain in respect of anything else: if people accept treatment without paying for it, it is just as bad as calling out a plumber and then refusing to pay him. Moreover, we might feel that, if people choose not to buy insurance, or not to buy healthcare at all, they still have a right in principle to access it — they have simply chosen not to exercise their right. Being *denied* the right is problematic, but the only person doing any denying in this picture is the would-be patient himself. Similarly, I have a right to get my drains unblocked, and my failure to call out the plumber does not diminish that right: it just means that I am not exercising it.

And yet there is a clear problem with this sort of picture. For it is obvious that, if I don't want to call out a plumber, I still could have a go at solving my problem myself. With a plunger, a set of tools and a little common sense, anyone could have a fairly good go at shifting the blockage or performing basic plumbing tasks. The same applies if my reason for not calling out the plumber is that I cannot afford to avail myself of his services, and also if there is no plumber nearby whom I can call: there is still nothing to stop me trying to fix the problem (and, anyway, we all have an incentive to make sure that we are not completely reliant on professionals whom we will have to pay). But when it comes to health, things are different. While anyone may choose to forego any treatment, if the reason that a person does not buy treatment or health insurance is that he cannot afford it, it will not do to shrug, sigh and tell him that he must therefore try to solve his problem for himself. There is no medical equivalent of DIY.

But this suggests that the right to healthcare is, in at least some respect, and despite first appearances, different from the right to buy other goods and services. If you have the right to healthcare, and if that healthcare requires private provision, and if you lack the means to buy private insurance, then your right turns out, at most, to have been purely formal. But a right that is purely formal is no such thing: for all the good that it will do them, we might just as well tell people that they have a right to walk to Venus. It is not really, of course, that your right has been *violated* by your not being able to access healthcare — noone is actively preventing access; but, still, for there to be a system in which that to which you have a right is inaccessible is for there to be a problem. What this means in practice is that if there is a meaningful human right to healthcare, we have a very good reason to expect that, at the very least, treatment such as is necessary for a reasonably tolerable life of a reasonable duration should be free at the point of receipt.

(I am ignoring here cases that might find an analogy in my perfect happiness not to have my drains unblocked when my slovenliness means that someone else is made to suffer: here, the state might properly intervene to force me to have the work done, though the question would not be one of my right to access plumbing, but of others' rights not to have inconvenience inflicted. In a world with only private medical care, the state might be entitled to make sure that I did not spread my contagion; and while the bill would be footed by the state in the first instance, if my illness reached its present state because of my negligence, it would presumably have the right to seek repayment from me. But note that, in this sort of case, we would not really be talking about a right to healthcare *as such*; we would be talking about others' rights not to be put in a position in which they need health care to begin with, and a concomitant obligation on my part either to accept a cure or to be locked away in a sanatorium where I can endanger noone else.)

Diversion: The Appeal to Justice

Parenthetically, the point can be bolstered by an appeal to justice or fairness. For we might well think that it offends against justice if a situation obtains under which only some people can get hold of something that everyone is supposed to be able to claim by right. If we can show that there is an unjust distribution of something to which all putatively have a right, we can use that to mount an argument against the system that allows that distribution to obtain and a secondary argument in favour of another system.

Now, private health insurance might simply not be an option for some people: maybe they were born with a congenital defect of some sort, or a genetic vulnerability to some kinds of disease, or something of the like. We can assume that insurers would have a disincentive to cover them—it makes much better business sense to provide health insurance to those who have a genetic inheritance that primes them for a long, active and healthy life. Thus, if I was an insurer, I might well want to make sure that my female clients are not carriers of the BRCA-1 gene, or that, if they are, they pay higher premiums; this is because the gene is associated with a raised risk of breast cancer, and clients with an increased susceptibility to cancer are likely to prove costlier to me than those without the susceptibility. (In just the same way, I might want to charge higher motor insurance premiums to inexperienced drivers with powerful cars.) And there might be some people to whom I would choose not to sell any insurance at all. Similarly, health providers would be foolish if they were to do anything other than charge more to those patients whose conditions were the most serious or demanding in terms of treatment and follow-up; those whose conditions are fairly transient and who are generally healthy, by contrast, are likely to need comparatively little attention for many conditions, and so will have to pay less. And this means that healthcare may be out of the reach of some people who suffer from "expensive" conditions.

If healthcare and health insurance was a matter of private contract, it would be odd to suppose that care providers or insurers could be denied the right to choose to whom they wanted to offer their services, for a contract into which one has no choice but to enter is not really a contract at all. A person might find, then, that he has an ostensible right to healthcare or insurance but that noone is willing to provide it; paradoxically, it might be that a person might find that he has limited access to healthcare *just because* he's the sort of person who is most likely to make use of it—this point is sometimes expressed as the "double jeopardy" problem. It is rational for me not to sell you health insurance because you're unhealthy, but it hardly seems fair to you.

We might want to bite this bullet and commiserate with the people who fall through the net without thinking that we have to do much to remedy such an instance of market failure. But adopting this line would mean moving away from the claim that healthcare is something to which we might have a right simply by virtue of being human and towards something more conditional. If we remain committed to the idea of healthcare as something to which a person has a fundamental right, we ought to be uncomfortable with the idea that a person might legitimately be unable to access healthcare, and bemused by the notion that the thing that prevents his access to healthcare is precisely his need for it. If we think that healthcare is a right, market failure might strike us as a reasonable explanation for a person's medical disenfranchisement, but it will not count as much of an excuse.

Part of the problem here is that the factor that makes some people less attractive to insurers is not under their control: if you have a genetic propensity to disease, this is hardly something for which you can be said to be responsible and so it seems unfair to disenfranchise you medically. Similar considerations might apply when we consider the situation of some other people in a world with only private healthcare provision. For example, providers of healthcare and health insurance might find that they have a disincentive to take on smokers or the obese as clients. Certainly, people have more control over smoking or obesity than they do over their genetic inheritance, so the problem is perhaps not so great here. But, to the extent that continued smoking is attributable to predisposition to addiction, or that obesity is attributable to having been lumbered with a particular metabolism or lack of willpower, none of which is entirely within the control of the individual, it looks as though all these situations describe cases in which a person might find that his right to healthcare is not all that powerful for reasons that are not within is power to alter, and which therefore clash with certain basic beliefs that we may have regarding fairness.

Other factors beyond a person's control that may have an impact on his ability to pay for private healthcare provision could include an injury that limits his capacity for work—remember that in this minimal world, there is no public welfare provision—or simply being a child with parents unable or too feckless to pay for cover. In all these cases, it would seem that there is something disquieting about a system in which some people do not have healthcare not because they have chosen to spend their money on other things, but simply because they have been unfortunate in their genetic inheritance, choice of parents, or something like that. The sense that something has gone wrong here may well reflect an appeal to certain commonsense standards of justice or fairness. It seems wrong to suppose that a person might not be able to claim his apparent right to healthcare because of these considerations; people ought not to be debarred from taking full advantage of that to which they have a right because of factors over which they have no control.

But what is the intellectual backing behind commonsense claims concerning justice? Aristotle's principle of justice is that we ought to treat equals equally, and unequals unequally according to that inequality (see Aristotle, 1992, 1242b14ff on this theme). In one sense, the difference in treatment is perfectly in keeping with some of the facts about the differences between people. On the other hand, though, if we think that healthcare is a human right, the relevant fact is common to those who can and those who cannot access healthcare: they are human. So this might explain our disquiet.

Another possible explanation for our disquiet might be suggested by adverting to a simplified version of the account that John Rawls

(1921–2002) spells out in detail in his *Theory of Justice*. One of the ways in which we might test whether a society is just is to imagine ourselves into the place of a randomly chosen member of that society. Naturally, each of us would want to occupy a place that was maximally well provided for, but we might also admit that inequality *per se* is not a problem (since we might all be better off in a world in which people have economic incentives to haul themselves up the social ladder — incentives that would be lacking in a strictly egalitarian world — we would be rational to allow for inequality), and that it does not conflict with justice for some to be worse off than others. Still, if we would find the position of the worst off intolerable, this would provide a hint that the society under scrutiny had a justice deficit for as long as it offered no remedy. And it seems unlikely that a rational person concerned for his own welfare would be willing to countenance life in a society in which he had no means to access at least basic healthcare, especially if he had been told that that healthcare was something to which he had a right (although he might equally well treat this last piece of information as little more than a joke).

Hence a society in which at least basic healthcare is potentially out of some people's reach is one that is less just than it might be. And since a sense of justice is central to many people's feelings about morality, it would seem to follow that such an apparently unjust system is something morally problematic. Therefore, again, it looks as though the moral demand is created for at least some healthcare the availability of which is independent of the ability to pay — that is, which is free at the point of delivery. In a well-ordered society, we would seem to need some way at least to paper over the social cracks and contingencies.

From the Right to Healthcare to State Provision

The point is that, if we think that there's a serious right to healthcare, and since the idea of a right that is not serious does not make all that much sense, it would seem to be inescapably the case that there is a moral reason for there to be at least a system of basic healthcare that is free at the point of delivery.

There is one line of objection with which we ought to deal at this point. Some might argue that there is nothing paradoxical about a situation in which we admit a right to healthcare but countenance some people not having access thereto. After all, there are many situations in which we might have a right to something without having to be able to access it. Each of us has the right to marry, for example. This means that noone has the right to forbid one person from marrying another person when both consent and neither is violating relevant bigamy laws. But accepting that there is a right to marry does not mean that any person has to be willing to marry us: it makes perfect sense to imagine a person who has a *right* to marry but who is, for whatever reason, simply not a person to whom anyone would want to get married. But the fact that a person cannot find anyone to marry him does not indicate that he has any less of a right to get married, and a right to marry does not imply a right to *be* married. *Mutatis mutandis*, the same might apply with a right to healthcare: a right to buy health insurance does not imply a right to be insured, and a right to healthcare does not imply a right to be cared for: in both cases, if noone is willing to provide the service you want, that is just too bad. The fact that a person cannot find anyone willing to provide health insurance would not, we might claim, dent her right to healthcare, notwithstanding what the previous argument suggests.

People influenced by *Anarchy, State and Utopia* by Robert Nozick (1938–2002) might argue in this way. It is arguably unfair that some people are unmarriageable, but it is not necessarily unjust; and whatever rights-based appeal there might be in respect of marriage goes no further than a right not to be forced into marriage. Under this libertarian account, rights are negative—they simply stop others interfering with your life. By extension, Nozickian libertarians are likely to dismiss the idea that there is a positive right to healthcare: at most, there is a negative right not to be made ill by others' deliberate actions.

Yet, since this chapter is concerned with what we should think *if* there were a right to healthcare, as the NHS claims, rather than whether there is a right to healthcare, we need only to pay as much attention to the analogy as it takes to foreclose it. (We shall meet Nozick again in the next chapter.) The marriage analogy can be dismissed simply by pointing out that *if* there is a right to marry, there must be a right to marry *someone*; and if there is no right to marry *someone*, there can be no right to marry. Therefore there is no right to be married after all (although there might still be a right not to be *prevented* from marrying, which is a little different). But the analogy with healthcare is misleading, and so perhaps tells us less than we might think. Certainly, *if* we think that there is a human right to healthcare, there is a corresponding right to access it. If there is no right to access, then there is no right to healthcare. But since (*ex hypothesi*) there is a right to healthcare, there must be a right to access it.

Yet even if accepting that there is such a thing as a right to healthcare implies that at least basic non-elective healthcare should be free at the point of delivery, we are not yet in a position to say that there ought to be an NHS, or even that it ought to fall to the state to provide healthcare. That is the next step.

The private sector is commonly thought to be the fee-charging sector, but there is no reason at all why we should regard such an equation as valid. After all, charities and benevolent funds could equally well count as private sources of healthcare, and we could look towards the charitable and benevolent parts of the private sector to provide the healthcare to which we apparently have a right. But, of course, there is still something not quite right about relying on charities and private benevolence to provide that to which we apparently have a right.

For one thing, we have to confront the very practical point that there is nothing to guarantee the capacity of such bodies to satisfy the demand for even basic healthcare. It is entirely plausible that their capacity would soon be exhausted. There is no shortage of examples of charities falling short of that which they want to achieve, both within and without the healthcare sector. Particularly pertinent examples are provided by those organisations that *sought* to provide free healthcare for the needy but which often could not afford to meet their own aims; not least among these examples is that set by the Royal Free Hospital in London. As its name implies, this institution was founded with the aim of providing free medical care. But, having been pushed close to bankruptcy, it was forced in the 1920s to ask patients to contribute what they could towards the cost of their treatment; it could not afford to carry the burden when it relied for funding on third parties. Of course, the very neediest might not have been asked to contribute anything (if what they could afford was nothing) — but the point is that institutions that aim to provide free healthcare are admirable, but may very well not be able to sustain the weight of the expectations they carry.

As well as this practical problem, there is a problem in principle with private beneficence. The point about charities or private benevolent institutions is that they are set up voluntarily. To this extent, their existence is supererogatory, and it is up to the founder (and, perhaps, the donors) to decide who benefits. But this means that there is little guarantee that the right kind of private institution will be founded or funded. I might set up a charity to offer relief from a certain condition or to a certain class of person — for example, I might be concerned to provide for the welfare of old philosophers, or of migraine sufferers — but this would be of no help to sailors forced out of work by polio, and the fact that I am willing to set up *an* institution to provide healthcare does not mean that I have an obligation to make its provision universal. Hence it is entirely possible that, while private institutions could make a contribution towards the provision of the healthcare to which we ostensibly have a right, not only is it the case that they cannot be relied upon to do any more; it is also the case that we would be in error if we were to expect more. In practice, and without impropriety, the reach of charities and private benevolent institutions is limited.

Citing this kind of point gives us a reason to think that the public sector ought to have something to do with the provision of healthcare if that healthcare is a right. It is at this point, then, that a supposition that there might be a right to healthcare begins to take on a concrete form as a demand that there should be a *public* health system of at least some minimal scope. Inasmuch as it is the state that provides the most obvious manifestation and representation of the public sector, it follows naturally from this that it is up to the state to guarantee at least minimal healthcare.

The suggestion that it is the public sector that provides the backstop of any rights that we have to healthcare has a number of attractive features. For one thing, the public sector — certainly when it is manifested in the form of the state or when the state is the default administrator of the public sector — has more resources at its disposal than the private. Of course, it is undeniable that states do go effectively bankrupt on occasion, and that their ability to provide healthcare is not absolutely reliable. But they are (on the face of it) much less likely than private institutions to suffer from a paralysing lack of liquidity. In the most simple and pragmatic terms, it looks as though, at the worst, the state might well be better fit than any of the alternatives to make sure that we get the healthcare to which we apparently have a right.

The idea that there is a moral argument for the involvement of the public sector (via the state) in the provision of healthcare also has the attraction that it avoids the problem that arose out of the limited scope of private institutions. For if something is a right but we are unable to get access to that thing, there would seem to be room to suppose that something is morally awry. If I have a right to something, that right ought to be bankable. But it would be odd to suppose that I might demand that someone set up a benevolent institution: my belief that whatever it is that would be provided by the foreseen institution would be something to which I had a right would not reduce this oddity. By contrast, there is nothing nearly so odd about making a similar demand of the state—especially if we think that part of the job of the state is to guarantee our human rights. In other words, if there is a right to healthcare and we are fortunate enough to live in a part of the world with a functioning public sector, we might well feel that that public sector, through the agencies of the state, is the proper backstop for our rights. After all—what would we make of a state that refused to acknowledge that people's rights come within its purview? And even if there is no functioning public sector, we might feel that any government ought to move to provide things like basic welfare for those whom it sought to govern to the extent that it is able.

It is entirely consonant with this kind of view to point out that, in a state that had no healthcare provision at all, we might hope that a charity would be able to intervene, and if none could, we would think this deeply regrettable; but if the state refused to make this provision (assuming, for the moment, that it was able), or if it did nothing to clear the way for the effective discharge of whatever private benevolence or private insurance was on offer, we would not think it regrettable: we would think it *blameable*. (This point harks back to my earlier claim about there still being a place for the state to act as a regulator in those worlds with only privately-provided medical cover.) Similarly, if a charity could no longer provide healthcare—and even if its trustees decided that they were no longer interested in providing what they had offered before—we would find this regrettable; but if the government of a country with a health service decided that it would abolish all public health provision the better to provide tax cuts, we would probably think that its behaviour was blameable, on the basis that noone ought to be medically disenfranchised. Again, the point is that, if there is a right to healthcare, we would think it bankable; and we would expect it to be bankable against the state (*qua* agent of the public sector) in a way that it is not against private healthcare providers.

There is, then, room for, and some sort of need for, a willingness on the part of the public sector, though the agency of the state, to intervene in order to guarantee at least minimal healthcare if healthcare is something to which we have a human right. A failure to endorse this kind of claim would mean derogating from the idea that we can properly think of healthcare as being a human right; and this would mean derogating from claims made by such organisations as the NHS and the UN. Granted that details may have yet to be filled in, we seem to have at least the skeleton of an argument for a public health service provided by the state and funded by the taxpayer— for who else provides liquidity to the public sector?

(Contrariwise, if we think that healthcare is something that we can claim as a matter of civil right and *not* as a matter of human right, then the idea that it *ought* to fall to the state to provide it begins to look odd. It is, after all, in the gift of the polity to decide what our civil rights are. Thus, if we want to say that there ought to be a public health service free at the point of delivery and that the state ought to provide it, we cannot be appealing to civil rights. In effect, this means that, though we might say that such a health service ought to be provided as a matter of political expediency, this "ought" has no particular moral sense and so will not contribute to a *moral* defence of a body such as the NHS.)

The "national" bit in a term like "National Health Service" can be argued for on the basis that the chances are that our nascent public health service would be most easily and most efficiently adminis- tered if we had a reasonably integrated network of healthcare outlets than it would be if those outlets were provided *ad hoc*. For example, we might think that it makes more sense to have 10 MRI scanners in each county in fairly constant use rather than one in each of its 15 major towns that is left idle for a good deal of the time, and such a setup would require integration, at least on a regional level. Simi- larly, we might think that there is only need for one or two outlets for more specialised services in the whole country, and that therefore we would be better off having an integrated system for them—the need to cure some tropical diseases quite possibly would not be all that pressing on a city-by-city basis, but, throughout the population of the country, there might be a need for one or two centres with this speciality. I am, of course, simply pulling numbers out of the air here, but I am presently concerned to do nothing more than to offer an illustration of a principle. Equally, in the real world, practical concerns might get in the way—but the principle would remain. National administration of the public health system might very well be a good way—the best way—of organising things.

At the same time, an integrated spending strategy would seem to be required on the basis of another appeal to rights. For even if healthcare is a right, there is another right that people can claim, which is the right to property. Now, I have just been claiming that, on the assumption that healthcare *is* a human right (as both the NHS and the UN claim), it follows that it generates duties of provision that are bankable (at least in the last resort) against the public sector. *Qua* constituent part of the public, each *member* of the public is a constituent part of that backstop—and this means that another's right to healthcare is, in part, bankable against each of us, the taxpayers who provide liquidity to the public sector. But taxpayers have a right not to be taxed more heavily than is strictly necessary, since over-taxation represents a violation of their right to property. (This point is adopted and exploited by Nozickians.) The taxpayers who foot the bill of each member of the public's right to healthcare have a right of their own for the nascent public health service to be as light a burden as possible. Accommodating such a right requires exploitation of economies of scale: again, national administration looks to be in order if (as seems likely) and to the extent that it would allow for the maximally efficient provision of a public health service.

Rights and Duties

At this point, it is worth making a quick point about the balance of rights and duties in the picture. It would appear that appeals to a right to healthcare have the upshot of making it the responsibility of the public sector, and therefore of the constituent members of the public, to provide the means to accommodate this right. The right seems to have generated a duty.

Of course, it is a commonplace that rights come alongside duties, and claims of this nature frequently get made by contributors to politics and news programmes. The contributors are right. However, they are frequently mistaken about *why* they are right.

What the contributors tend to want to say is that a person cannot claim a right to this or that without admitting that they have certain duties as well—they envisage a *quid pro quo* under which one "earns" rights or the guarantee of rights through the discharge of duties. If we are talking about political or civil rights, this claim may be true: there is nothing too incoherent about a monarch granting a person the right to drive geese over London Bridge in return for duties of loyalty, for example. But if we are talking about *human* rights, and if we take the idea of a human right seriously, the picture is somewhat different. If there is such a thing as a human right, it seems abundantly clear that it is the sort of thing that one can have without taking on duties. This is obviously the case with infants, of whom we tend to think as having at least some rights (such as a right to be fed and not to be killed or molested) but who cannot plausibly have any duties. Indeed, *anyone's* right not to be killed or molested is not dependent on their having accepted duties. If we think that I have a human right to something, and/or that this right is fundamental, the very fact that it is fundamental counts as a strong suggestion that it is dissociable from any duties that I might have. Granted that I do have some duties but I fail to discharge them, my fundamental rights would be unaffected. In this sense, possession of a right does not imply having a duty.

On the other hand, if I have an entitlement to something as a matter of human right, and this right is enforceable, then it does generate some kind of a duty — but it is a duty imposed on other people. Minimally, it means that they have a duty to respect that right — which is as much as to say that they have a duty not to prevent me from accessing that to which I have the right unless they can provide a compelling argument for my right's having been trumped — but it may mean that they have a more substantial duty. So, for example, your decision to brick up your front door is perfectly acceptable unless I have a right to walk through it, in which case you have a duty of some kind not to. Your right to property means that I cannot knock down your house, unless — as Locke admits (Locke, 1960, para 159) — it is on fire and the fire cannot be put out and presents a threat to my house too (because your rights over your fire-damaged property might be trumped by my right not to have my hitherto undamaged property damaged).

Now, if healthcare is one of those things to which one might have a *human* right, then it will generate duties — but one does not "earn" the right to healthcare by virtue of contributions to the public sector. Instead, the tab for this right is picked up by the public sector. Bearing in mind one of the myths of the modern state — that there is, or at least ought to be, no appreciable distinction between government and people — will show how the duties fall upon us, *qua* constituent members of the public: presumably, the moral proximity of the people and the state means that the people can share the credit for the state's successes and exploit its advantages, but must also share its responsibilities not so much as a matter of reciprocity as because any alternative is incoherent.

In this case, then, it so happens that the rights-holders are the same as the duty-holders. But the principle that rights and duties are basically separable remains.

But we ought to return to the main thrust of the argument: it would seem to appear that the moral framework has been provided for, in the first place, a *public* health service, and, in the second, something like a *national* public health service. In other words, whatever gaps need to be filled in, we can see the rough outline of a rights-based argument for something very like the NHS.

Beyond the NHS: What Public?

In actual fact, though, the success of a moral argument for a public heath service based on an appeal to human rights does not generate all that strong a moral argument for a national health service so much as it generates an argument for a *trans*national health service. For although everyday talk about the public sector tends to treat "the public sector" as "that which the state provides", it does not follow that the public sector is in any way *defined* by the remit of the state. Certainly, in the sense that I have been using it, the term "public sector" simply indicates everything that cannot be limited to specific and identifiable agents, and so those public responsibilities and duties that fall to the state do so as a matter of expediency (to the extent that the state *represents* and *acts on behalf of* the public sector), but nothing more. Allowing that "the state" is more-or-less interchangeable with "the nation" in this context—which is not much of an allowance given that extant public health services are arranged on an state-by-state basis rather than on an appeal to "the nation" in any other sense—the point translates.

But having disallowed the use of the state to define the public sector and said instead that the public sector is simply that which is not limited to specific agents, it looks as though I am committed to saying that whatever duties befall the public sector thereby befall everyone and noone in particular—and this statement is too nebulous really to carry much moral weight. I can only admit that the first part of this charge is fair: the duties that befall the public sector *do* befall everyone and noone in particular. In fact, though, it would be odd to admit anything else. However, this does not mean that the position I have adopted is morally impotent.

To see why, it is worth spending some time reexamining the notion of a human right. If I have a right to something or to do something—say, a right to free speech—then it will generate a duty. As I have argued, the duty that it generates falls on others. In this example, others have a duty to allow me to say pretty much what I want to say (although there might be restrictions on where I can say it — hence the freedom of speech does not mean that it is OK for me to shout "Fire!" in a crowded theatre, or to gossip through the performance).

What is important, though, is that, when we are talking about those others who have a duty not to interfere with that to which I have a right, it does not matter who they are. If free speech is something to which I can lay claim as a matter of human right, the corresponding duty is something that falls on everyone and noone in particular; this is exactly what makes it a public duty. And while I might expect the government of each country to take measures as far as possible to guarantee the right (perhaps by enshrining it in law), the moral point would be that *anyone* who tried to forbid my saying what I had to say would have violated my right to say it, and, to that extent, wronged me. Therefore if the government or people of some country or other tried to silence me, they would have wronged me; and on the basis of the claim that free speech is a human right, not just a political or civil right, it would not matter whether I was a citizen of that country. If free speech is a human right, it ought to apply equally well *in* each and every state, just because, *qua* human right, it is something that obtains "above" the level of the state. (Of course, this does not mean that anyone has to provide the means for me to make my point — it simply means that, if I have the means, I ought not to be prevented from making use of them.)

Translated to healthcare, similar arguments can be made. Allowing that healthcare is a human right, that a notional human right that cannot be claimed by someone turns out not to be a human right at all, and that it is up to the public sector to guarantee that right, then the country of which I happen to be a citizen cannot really make much of a difference in respect of that right. I may look to the state in my home country to guarantee that right, but this is not the same as the state in my home country being the *fons et origo* of my right. (If it were, it would begin to look like a civil, rather than a human right.) As with free speech, a human right to healthcare is something that obtains "above" the level of the state.

Now, *qua* constituent members of the public sector, we are the guarantors of our neighbours' right to healthcare, and this remains the case even though the responsibility is not one that we have chosen to adopt. This is not because our neighbour is our compatriot or fellow-citizen: it is because he is human; and the upshot of this is that if compatriotism and citizenship do not have much to do with the duties that our neighbours' rights impose on us, they are supranational. In other words, if we think that access to healthcare is a human right and that the guarantor of that right is everyone who counts as a member of the public, and since everyone does count as a member of the public, the guarantor of the right will be everyone.

But this means, in turn, that, for the same reasons that we have a duty to act as a co-guarantor of our compatriots' healthcare, so we have a duty to act as a co-guarantor of the healthcare of everyone whom we acknowledge as human. For it does make sense to talk in terms of there being a "global public" of which we are all members — remember that I have already claimed that the state is founded in a public sector that it merely represents and regulates, rather than *vice versa* — no less sense, in fact, than it does to talk in terms of there being a national public from which a state might derive its legitimacy and to which it might owe its responsibilities. If the NHS is founded on the claim that healthcare is a human right, for it not to act in some way towards guaranteeing access to healthcare for every human, or for it not to present itself as simply a part of a wider network of welfare institutions around the world, is an indication that it is — or we are — guilty of muddled thinking. Muddled thinking, though, might not be *wrong* in any serious moral sense, but it is indefensible. (I shall return to considerations of the place of the NHS in respect of wider networks later.)

The conclusion that, as constituent members of the global public, we all have a duty incumbent upon us to act as joint guarantors of all humans' right to healthcare is startling. But if healthcare is a human right, I believe that it is inescapable. What it does not mean is that we have a duty as individuals to make cash donations to medical charities — another argument would be needed to generate this kind of claim — but it does mean that the fact that a person cannot access healthcare is something for which we cannot say we have no responsibility. If someone has no access to healthcare, and if healthcare is something that he can claim as a matter of right, that should be a source of moral worry to us, irrespectively of whether or not he is a compatriot, just as the impossibility of free speech in a police state ought to be a worry for us if we think that free speech is a human right.

The difference between a right to healthcare and a right to free speech is that it is easier to do something about guaranteeing the former than the latter. If someone's right to speak is threatened, there might be little that we, as members of the public, can do except agitate, and get governments to agitate on our behalf. But, with respect to healthcare, it is possible for the global public sector to intervene. Now, there might seem to be a problem here. In practical terms, it tends to be up to the state to guarantee human rights on behalf of the public sector — it is not so much that it is the best fit body for the task, as that it is the only body. There is no transnational analogue of the state. However, there is a couple of counterpoints that can be put to this. In the first place, if the responsibility for guaranteeing people's rights lies with the public, then the fact that there *is* no presently-existing agency that can serve whatever demands might properly be made is less important than the answers to the twin questions of whether there *ought* to be and whether there *can* be such a body. The answer to the question of whether there ought to be is given in what I have just been arguing, and I have no wish to labour the point. The question of whether there *can* be is, as far as I can see, dependent on two factors: logistics and public willingness.

The logistical concerns need not worry us. It is patently obvious that it is possible for there to exist perfectly viable transnational state-like organisations. The various agencies of the United Nations provide ample evidence for this: granted political willingness on the part of the constituent members of the UN, bodies such as the WHO, the World Food Programme and UNICEF are capable if implementing transnational healthcare policies in a state-like manner. Some governments may (for some reason) seek to isolate themselves from foreign intervention of this sort — but this looks as though they might be seeking to deprive their citizens of the healthcare to which we think they have a right; and this means they are wronging their citizens. A government that wrongs its citizens, though, might be the kind of government whose policies we have a moral reason to oppose, ignore, or seek to undermine.

What is left is a set of worries about willingness. But willingness, too, need not bother us all that much. If we are talking about human rights, the fact that it falls to the public sector to act as the guarantor of those rights is something in which it has no choice. If a person has a human right to something, others simply have an inescapable duty to take account of that right, and their willingness to do so is not an issue. We would not say that a person has a human right to free speech but that it rests on others' willingness to *let* him speak freely: we would say instead that he has a right to free speech and that it is up to others simply to accommodate it. (By contrast, public willingness to act as a guarantor *is* important in respect of civil rights, because, for them, the removal of the guarantee will mean effectively that the right has evaporated or been transformed into more of a privilege—which can, of course, be withdrawn.) Thus if healthcare really is a human right, our willingness to stand as guarantors is neither here nor there.

At the same time, it might well be the case that, for example, a British person might properly look to the British state, a German person to the German state, and a Malian person to the Malian state to act as the direct provider of healthcare. But this does not mean that he can look no further should his home country be unable or unwilling to provide. After all, I have already suggested that there would be something odd if, faced with a child who happens to be born to parents who are unwilling or unable to provide healthcare, we were to say that he has a right to healthcare while doing nothing more than to offer commiserations about his inability to access it. Such an attitude would indicate that we did not take his notional right seriously. Exactly the same rationale forces us to admit that, if a person happens to live in a part of the world where the government is unwilling or unable to provide him with at least minimal healthcare, and if we think that healthcare is a human right, it is inadequate simply to commiserate with him about *his* misfortune. We have to admit that his right, if right it be, is bankable against the public sector —which includes us foreigners.

Bluntly, if there is a human right to healthcare, it is presumably a right that all humans have. A body like the NHS goes some way to meeting this right. Still, if it is a human right to healthcare that motivates the existence of an NHS or corresponding bodies within a state, it ought also to be the case that this national service is seen as nothing more than a part of a larger public health service. An appeal to human rights will not generate, and ought not to be thought of as capable of generating, a *national* health service *per se*.

If public willingness to contribute to provide access to healthcare on a global scale *is* an issue, and if the public sector has a right to decide that it will not guarantee such access, then healthcare turns out not to have been a human right after all. But if we were to choose to reject the idea that healthcare might be a human right and the correspondingly generated argument for a transnational health service, we would, as far as I can see, by the same token have ditched any moral argument for there being an NHS at all that sought its basis in an appeal to rights.

If it is an appeal to merely civil rights that does the moral work, the NHS would be better grounded—although, trivially, it would have to rethink some of the claims it makes for itself. Nevertheless, there might be other reasons to think that, when it comes to providing welfare to others, concentrating on the national might represent something of a moral error. Even if a free public health service is a civil right, there might still be a moral duty to provide free healthcare transnationally — this will be the theme of the next chapter — and the right might be trumped by other factors — this will be the theme of the chapter after that.

Chapter 3

Public Health and Duty

It would appear, as things stand, that we can give a reasonably good argument in defence of the claim that, if there is a right to healthcare, and if that right really is a human right rather than simply a civic right, we have a moral reason to provide a public health service whose reach is transnational; put another way, we have no particular reason to provide a *national* health service. Providing a national health service represents a way for us to begin to accommodate people's putative human right to healthcare, but if we are concerned to accommodate those rights as fully as possible — which seems to be demanded by the supposition that they are human rights at all — we will quickly find we have exhausted what can be provided by a national health service.

On some accounts of rights, though, there is still room for dispute about the provision of a public health service. Those who want to defend healthcare's status as something to which we have a human right or an entitlement — it does not matter for the moment whether that right or entitlement comes from membership of a community, or whether it's something more basic like a human right — might face an attack from one of two fronts.

One line of attack is constituted by the simple denial that there is a right to healthcare, at least inasmuch as that right is supposed to be fundamental and irreducible to other considerations. Such an attack might be mounted as a part of a wider sceptical claim about human rights *tout court*. Whatever else we might say about the provision of healthcare, we might have no right to have it provided for the simple reason that we have no relevant rights.

Another line of attack that might be used against a rights-based argument for a public health service is to turn it against itself. Some people might want to argue against the provision of a public health service not because we have no *right* to healthcare — or, at least, not primarily because we have no such right — but rather because, whatever rights we do have to healthcare, they are simply less important than other rights, and these other rights cancel out the healthcare right. In other words, the claim would be that there is no *significant* or *overriding* right to healthcare; and we could—if we were feeling concessive—make this claim while still allowing that there is a *weak* right to healthcare.

But how might such an argument work? One approach would be to exploit a line suggested by Robert Nozick's account of justice. We have already seen how the account of justice offered by John Rawls might be put to work in favour of the public provision of welfare services. Nozick's account of justice differs significantly; for while (at risk of oversimplifying affairs) Rawls is concerned with justice as the "end point" of social policy, Nozick is concerned to provide a procedural account of justice. He is not so much concerned by how the end picture looks, as by how we arrive at it. This means, in passing, that a world with massive inequality need not be thought of as unjust. For as long as people get what they get without infringing others' rights, there is no injustice in any particular distribution. But what are those rights?

For Nozick, an important consideration is the right to live one's life in a manner as free from others' interference as possible. Of course, people might volunteer to curb their own activities in all kinds of ways, but noone has a right to interfere in my life without a very good reason. Among the rights that we might have is the right not to be made ill; but this is not the same as saying that there is a right to healthcare. I can, if I choose, take vitamin supplements and wear a surgical mask when I go outside, for such is my right. I also have grounds for complaint if you recklessly sneeze on me: such grounds are compatible with my right not to be made ill or to suffer any form of needless inconvenience; however, if I did become ill, I would not from that fact alone be able to say that I had any right to treatment. Perhaps you might owe me compensation for having sneezed on me, but even that isn't so much to do with my right to healthcare as with your already having violated my right not to be sneezed on recklessly.

Now, the problem with claiming that a right to healthcare generates a moral argument for a publicly funded health service is that it means that individuals, inevitably, will be forced into contributing towards that scheme. Public spending means that a portion of my labour will be appropriated by the public pot; after all, it is funded, one way or another, by taxation. But taxation, Nozick thinks, is on a par with forced labour, and that is a violation of my liberty. He claims that,

> [i]f people force you to do certain work, or unrewarded work, for a certain period of time, they decide what you are to do and what purposes your work is to serve apart from your own decisions (Nozick, 1974, p 172)

and this looks something akin to slavery. Living in a world in which a part of the product of our work is taken from us by anyone else — even the community — indicates a shift from a classical liberal picture of self-ownership to one in which one person, or the community as a whole, can have at least partial property rights in other people. For Nozick, this is unacceptable; thus, he thinks, "the state may not use its coercive apparatus for the purpose of getting some citizens to aid others" (*ibid*, p ix).

The point is that, if we care about freedom — as most of us do — then this might well trump any notional right to healthcare. The charge is that hackneyed redistributive claim that justice involves giving to people according to their need is all well and good, except for the fact that it requires forcing people to contribute. This is a violation of their rights. By contrast, not to force contributions for the sake of healthcare makes noone worse off than they otherwise would have been: it simply means that we are not making them any healthier. This might be a bad thing, of course; and if it is a bad thing, we are free to do something about it. But the fact that we're free to do something about it means that our rights aren't violated when we do so. Our choosing to give away a certain percentage of our earnings to others is massively different from those others being allowed access to our bank accounts so that they can take the same percentage from us without regard for our preferences.

Still, the idea that we are free to help others would be difficult to deny; moreover, we might want to go further, and suggest that we have a duty to do so. As we shall see in the coming pages, it is possible to come up with an account of duties that is not in conflict with freedom and so not in conflict with concerns that we might have to protect people's rights. If it can be got to work argumentatively, we might be able to provide an account of how there is a duty to contribute to a public health service even though we might still think that noone has any serious right to healthcare. As we go, the clear suggestion will be that, if there is an obligation to set up a public health service, then it ought to be transnational in scope, for there is no clear reason to suppose that political boundaries impose limits on the duties that we owe to each other.

Whereas some duties are grounded in others' rights and are, in a sense, nothing more than the footprint of those rights, not all duties have to be conceptualised in this way; and the kind of duty that I shall consider in this chapter is different from the "footprint duty" I mentioned in the last because it is a duty of precisely the sort that is not predicated on others having rights of the correct sort. I might think that I have a duty to give a certain portion of my income to charity where possible, but this does not commit me to the thought that any recipient of charitable *largesse* has a right bankable against me for that contribution to be made. This was, of course, an important consideration in the discussion of private benevolence in the last chapter, where I pointed out that, even if there is a right to health-care, it would make little sense to demand of anyone that they set up a charitable institution as a means to guarantee this right.

As we shall see from this chapter, any scepticism that we have about rights, or about the scope of rights, will not suffice to warrant mutual indifference — we might still have duties to each other, some of which might be enforceable. (Not all duties are enforceable, by the way: I might have a duty to cultivate an unconditional positive regard for others, but it is hard to see how anyone could enforce this should I fail to discharge my duty.) If it is plausible to suppose that there are duties that we owe each other *a priori*, then we could allow at least the possibility that there is a duty to contribute to others' welfare without their having any corresponding right; and, having made that allowance, we could talk meaningfully about how we might go about discharging that duty in the real world. Should such a picture prove paintable, it would meet Nozickian worries about us having a right to property, but it could also (with the right details) still generate an argument for something looking very like a public health service based on an account of individuals' positive duties towards each other.

Duties without Rights

One argument for the establishment of something like a public health service would be based on an appeal to the duties that we owe to each other simply by virtue of being moral agents. The strongest argument in favour of there being such duties comes from the deontological tradition, the defining characteristic of which is the idea that one can describe moral duties in a "free standing" manner, without reference to the ends that one might want to achieve by one's actions. (Thus if you think that, say, adultery is just wrong and would remain so even if (a) highly enjoyable to the participants and (b) never having any deleterious consequences for anyone, you might be making an appeal to deontology.) But more consequentialist accounts of morality can also yield directives for action. Admittedly, some might squirm a little at the idea that consequentialism is compatible with appeals to duty in the strict sense: but the directives that it does generate look enough like duties to count as such for my purposes.

For consequentialists, the moral value of an action is a function of its consequences. The better an action's consequences, the more entitled we are to ascribe rightness to it; and we measure the goodness of its consequences in terms of welfare (understood in its loosest sense). For John Stuart Mill (1806–73), welfare claims always boiled down to claims about happiness: that an action tended to make us happy was an indication that it was optimific; and happiness was the *only* indication that an action was optimific (see Mill, 1998, ch. 4 for the argument on this). Other theorists might be willing to accommodate a wider conception of what contributes to the good: but the point is that it is contributions to the good that are important. To the extent that—when consequentialism is put into practice— contributing to the good is properly described as right, it is something that we ought to do. If, for consequentialist reasons, we ought to contribute to others' welfare, we can treat this as a duty.

Now, it does seem that there would be a good reason to suppose that the world would be a better place if we were more willing to contribute to others' welfare, and not just because the effects of such a concern rebound well on us (as would have to be the case to sustain an argument from self interest). For as long as the increase in welfare outweighed the sacrifice made by each contributor, there would be a moral reason to contribute. Admittedly, one of the problems with this kind of reasoning is that, however small the sacrifice *I* make, and however large the benefit I thereby bestow on you, it is inescapably the fact that I have little incentive to contribute. But this kind of objection might well misfire, for the picture here is one in which we have a moral reason to act for the general welfare and to discount our own: the world simply ends up as a better place that way—and optimising the state of the world is what concerns consequentialists like Mill. If we think that there might be a duty to contribute to the general welfare, the fact that, all told, we'd prefer not to is neither here nor there. The point is that private philanthropy based on

motives of beneficence can be taken as something that we ought to
contemplate and upon which we ought to act.

There are ways to talk about duties without appeals to consequence,
though. Famously, Immanuel Kant (1724–1804) — whose aim is to
give an account of morality that is purged of any empirical considerations, so that we can derive a conception of what is good in itself
— thinks that we have a duty to promote the welfare of humanity not
because of the obvious attraction that this must have for members of
humanity, but because framing a will to act in this way is demanded
by morality even without regard to the ends we hope to achieve
thereby. Kant tends to argue for his practical claims not so much by
saying directly that one must do this or that, but by pointing out that
any defence of *not* doing it would be unsustainable, and that is his
strategy here.

In the first place, Kant admits cheerfully enough that "[p]roviding
for oneself to the extent necessary just to find satisfaction in living
([to a point that includes] taking care of one's body [...]) belongs
among duties to oneself" and that, as long as we harm noone else,
matters could apparently be left in this state: "the maxim 'Everyone
for himself, God (fortune) for us all' seems to be the most natural
one" (Kant, 1996, 6:452). However, Kant wants to claim that, despite
appearances, we cannot leave matters in this state. For if a maxim is
to be found compatible with the laws of morality, it must apply uni-
versally: we must be able to picture a world in which all persons
behaved according to a given maxim not just as a matter of course,
but all the time. A world in which a maxim thus universalised undermines itself cannot truly reflect the demands of morality, Kant
thinks, because the demands of morality obtain without reference to
the who, the where and the why of the situation. ("We must," he
claims, "be able to will that a maxim of our action become a universal
law: this is the canon for morally estimating any of our actions."
(Kant, 1993, 4:424)) And the apparently natural maxim of self-interest to the exclusion of others, it is claimed, cannot be universalised;
therefore it cannot conform with the moral law.

It is worth quoting Kant's argument at length here:

> To be beneficent, that is, to promote according to one's means the
> happiness of others in need, without hoping for something in
> return, is everyone's duty.
>
> For everyone who finds himself in need wishes to be helped by
> others. But if he lets his maxim of being unwilling to assist others
> in turn when they are in need become public [i.e. generally
> accepted, rather than simply widely known — IB], that is, makes

this a universal permissive law, then everyone would likewise deny him assistance when he himself is in need, or at least would be authorised to deny it. Hence the maxim of self-interest would conflict with itself if it were made a universal law, that is, it is contrary to duty. Consequently the maxim of common interest, of beneficence towards those in need, is a universal duty of human beings ... (Kant, 1996, 6:453)

Kant's claim is not directly that willingness to help others is a moral duty: but if he can show that *unwillingness* to help others violates the (disinterested) laws of morality — and he thinks he can — he will have made the point indirectly. Beneficence is a duty, but not so much because it is good (which is the point at which consequentialists would think the argument complete) as because, like it or not, non-beneficence is morally ruled out. (It is worth noting, before going further, that the duty of beneficence is understood by Kant as a part of a wider duty of love to other human beings, which I shall denote with the word "philanthropy"; henceforward I shall, as the context demands, flit between the words "philanthropy" and "beneficence", but this does not mean that I am smuggling in a sense that is additional to that intended by Kant.) He makes substantially the same point about beneficence elsewhere: though mutual indifference could prevail as a law of nature — there is nothing paradoxical about the concept, however undesirable a world in which it was the rule — it is not possible for us to *will* that it should (see Kant, 1993, 4:423 and, less clearly, 4:430). Of course, a needy person's wish that others should offer him aid does not imply that those others ought automatically to grant his wishes, but this exactly is why Kant thinks that beneficence is only an *imperfect* duty: although it is not incoherent for us to *imagine* a world in which the putative duty is systematically violated, it would be paradoxical for us to *will* it.

Considerations of whether or not the argument as Kant puts it is wholly convincing need not detain us here (although we might suspect that Kant has raised a false dichotomy and that there is a perfectly tenable midpoint between attending to others' needs and scorning them). What matters is merely that an argument is produced the effect of which is to suggest that what we might call a "failure of beneficence" would violate a duty of some sort. Other deontological accounts might set about the task in other ways but can still offer us a reason to suppose that a failure of beneficence would indicate a failure to discharge our moral duties. Now, if we are convinced by such arguments, we may well find in them a moral reason to provide something like a public health service.

If beneficence is a duty, we might spin this out to mean that it is incumbent on us as relatively decent moral agents to make regular and tolerably frequent contributions to charities, benevolent institutions and so on. However, the potential criticism of such a would be that, in selecting our recipients in this way, we have in some manner derogated from our general duty of beneficence. Giving to specific good causes might be an *expression* of philanthropy, but it might equally not be, and it certainly is not a substitute. After all, it is possible for us to contribute to specific charitable institutions without being enormously philanthropic. For example, we might choose to give to a medical charity out of philanthropy, but we might also do so because the illness for which it provides treatment runs in our family, with the understandable result that we're motivated by a desire to make sure that we get the best treatment possible. If it is the second consideration that motivates us, it would fit alongside a general disdain for humanity without contradiction.

Even if this criticism is destined to fail, if our motivation to donate is based on a general philanthropy, rather than anything that is ends-directed, we ought not object to the donations that we make to charity being put towards any and all good ends: if it is philanthropy that motivates us, then some system in which all charities that aim to contribute to relief for the needy would get a share of our contributions, regardless of who those needy are and the provenance of their need, ought not to be objectionable to us. Perhaps we might even welcome such a system, as it would allow us to discharge our duty without having to worry that we were being distracted and our philanthropy perverted by our idiosyncratic concerns. A person's notional right to do with his wealth as he sees fit might appear to undermine this suggestion, except that the "as he sees fit" criterion may be in tension with the general beneficence demanded by duty. (We could, of course, give away with impunity a portion of what is left after the reasonable demands of beneficence had been satisfied.)

However, private philanthropy might not be the best way for us to discharge our duties: if it is the welfare of humanity that directs our actions and leads us to give a reasonable portion of our wealth to the needy, that motivation would not be distorted by a system under which a portion of our wealth was taken by the state for the sake of the needy (let's say in the form of a tax) and distributed as seen fit by the experts doubtless employed by the state. Certainly, this looks like a plausible enough upshot of the consequentialist approach: for if there were some organisation that could collect and pool the resources of the mass of private philanthropists, it would likely be able to exploit economies of scale and thereby wring every possible unit of welfare from the contributions made.

We might be worried that such a "philanthrotax" involves an infringement of the liberties the protection of which might have motivated a Nozickian challenge to public healthcare; indeed, it also looks like it might be a violation of the autonomy that is central to Kant's moral theory (see Kant, 1993, *passim*). The worry would be that even if we are prepared to swallow the claim that we *do* have duties to provide for others, it is still up to us to discharge those duties: noone has the right to force us to do what we ought. If we are drawn towards consequentialist reasoning, such a critique will not bother us unduly. It's the outcome that matters, and, while violating someone's freedom might well make a dent in the level of welfare in the world (unfree people leading, it is reasonable to assume, lives less good than those of the free), it would be warranted by the expected payoff; besides, there might be something optimific about a philanthrotax if it relieves people of the burden of having to take responsibility for their own beneficence.

Worries about freedom might loom larger in non-consequentialist accounts; but, even here, they would be unfounded. Part of the reason for this is that we might imagine a sophisticated philanthrotax system that allowed people to opt out. Exploiting such an opt-out might strike us as mildly villainous, but if a person chooses to act contrary to the demands of morality, then that is his affair. But even without an opt-out, there would not necessarily be a conflict between the philanthrotax and free philanthropy. The reason for this is suggested by Harry Frankfurt in a paper from 1969. Frankfurt argues here that the idea of acting freely does not depend on an agent's having a range of possible alternative actions. Roughly, the argument works like this: if someone puts a gun to my head and demands that I drink the coffee, for just as long as that was what I was going to do *anyway*, his presence has had no impact on me at all. It is only if I have no intention to drink the coffee that my freedom or right to do as I please is violated. Applied to this case, for as long as we were going to sacrifice a portion of our income *anyway*, being told that we have to do so adds nothing. A philanthrotax would only infringe my freedom if the other option open to me was to violate the demands of morality — which, being a reasonably decent sort of person, was not something I was contemplating.

Indeed, because such a system—the basic mechanics of the centralised system of welfare resource distribution that I outlined in the last chapter would bear being coopted by an argument that concentrates on duties with, at most, a few tweaks—would have the advantage of being able to maximise the efficiency with which the funds could be gathered and spent, we might expect a decent person to welcome a philanthrotax because it would maximise the impact of his philanthropy. It does not take too much of a leap of the imagination to see that the system being outlined looks very like a public welfare system: if we have an obligation to provide support, and the state can provide the means to administer this support efficiently and disinterestedly, then there cannot be much in the way of viable objection to the state having a role in the discharge of our duties of beneficence.

Public and National Health Services

Does this mean that we have what is needed to generate an argument for the provision of a public health service such as the NHS based on an appeal to duty? For reasons that are similar in tone to those that I produced in the arguments in the rights chapter, we could answer this by separating the arguments for a *public* health service from those for a *national* health service. As we shall see, the argument from duty gives a strong indication that the former would be better founded, morally speaking, than the latter.

The part of the argument that serves to promote a public health service would rely on the plausible assumption that a part of the requirement to aid the needy would involve providing for them at least minimal or emergency healthcare, since philanthropy aims at an increase in the welfare of humanity and health has a good claim to be a constituent part of that welfare. Just because the provision of such care would be provided under the impetus of a duty of philanthropy, it would not make much sense to say anything other than that it ought to be free at the point of delivery—after all, we would not think it quite right to suppose that a needy person should be willing to offer recompense beyond gratitude for our having reduced his need, and even then, to insist on gratitude would be churlish. At the same time, we might suppose that those who do not, strictly speaking, need the fruits of our beneficence would have an obligation to forego them; but such constraints on others' behaviour do not really militate against what is required of us—if we think that we have a duty of philanthropy or beneficence, we ought not to think it lessened by the possibility that unscrupulous people might exploit our virtue.

I think, too, that considerations such as the virtuous desire to see our philanthropy provide as much as possible generate a good reason to support its being mediated by a centrally-administered public health service rather than a collection of potentially rag-tag private philanthropic organisations, the extent of whose welfare provision might anyway turn out to be somewhat incomplete.

All the same, central administration is all well and good—but central to what? Granted that, as I argued in the last chapter, there is a tendency to equate the public sector with the state sector, this might lead us to assume that a public health service will be something like a national health service. But the argument in the last chapter should have uncoupled the two; and they remain uncoupled here. Hence talking about the public sector as a vector for our philanthropy will not automatically entitle us to treat a public health system interchangeably with a national health system. Moreover, the arguments in favour of the public provision of health services that I have presented are pretty indiscriminate. If philanthropy—love for humanity—is a duty, for example, it ought to follow from this that the recognition that someone is a human is sufficient to give them a certain place in our esteem; and if that philanthropy generates moral pressure for a public health system of some sort, then it would seem to follow that that system would be directed at humanity in a correspondingly indiscriminate manner. If we allow for these considerations, it begins to look as though we have provided—as with the argument from rights—an argument for a health system that may be administered by states, and so *de facto* nationally, but not for a *national* health service *as such*.

Similarly, if we are attracted by more consequentialist reasoning, we would still admit that we have an obligation to act in an optimific manner, and that this will give us a moral reason to act on behalf of whomever it is that will benefit the most from our actions. Very likely, this will mean concentrating our health system overseas. After all, the greatest improvement to humanity's lot will be provided by spending the welfare budget where it is likely to have the highest marginal value—and an extra million pounds wisely spent in western Europe will improve the lot of humanity, but not as much as it would if it was wisely spent in central Africa. So the argument, carried through consistently, seems to suggest that, if optimificity is our concern, there is a reason to resist any such thing as a national health service, except (again) insofar as states might well turn out to be the best local administrators of a transnational system. This kind of consideration will be important for the argument of chapter 4; for the remainder of this chapter, I shall concentrate on the implications of non-consequentialist arguments.

Moral Gravity

Allowing a duty of philanthropy or beneficence seems to lead to an argument for a transnational health service. But it is almost certain that we would be too hasty if we thought that the debate was therefore closed. For much of its cogency depends on the assumption that we ought to be impartial between persons: that, whatever duties we have, we have in respect of all persons equally. If it can be shown that moral impartiality is not required, or that some kind of partiality *is* required, the transnationalism of the last section will potentially fall into abeyance, and there will be scope to reintroduce an argument for a public health service organised on national grounds.

Certainly, the idea that our duties obtain in the same kind of way regardless of to whom it is that we owe them is plausible in a lot of cases—perhaps in most cases. Thus, for example, my duty not to kill, rape or steal from you is pretty constant, irrespective of who you are (with the possible exception of cases in which, say, killing you is self-defence proportional to the threat you represent, or in which I am a starving person who steals a loaf of bread from a bakery).

However, not all duties obtain equally. Whatever our "baseline" duties, there are some people who are more properly the objects of our concern than others. At the same time, even if everyone has the same rights, there need not be a problem with being more concerned by some people's rights than by others', and thereby feeling that the duties that those rights generate are different. Even if all people are morally equal, it does not follow that we owe them equal consideration.

How might this be? The point can be illustrated by an analogy. Imagine that, in orbit around a nearby star, is a planet that is exactly like Earth in every respect. Call this twin Earth "Twearth". Earth and Twearth, naturally, have the same gravitational mass. Nevertheless, it is obvious that Earth's gravity has a much greater effect on me than has Twearth's, just because of where each of them is and where I am. The point is that, even if each person has an equal moral status (a point so trivially true as not really to need argumentative support) and they therefore have a similar "moral gravity", it does not follow that the moral gravity of each person will have the same draw *on us*. Some people, some people's rights, and the duties that I owe to some, are just more important to me, just because of who they are and who I am.

Commonsense morality would seem to support the analogy. For example, a parent who thinks that her duties towards her own child are no different from those that she owes to others' children would quite properly be an object of moral criticism, or puzzlement at the very least, since we tend to think that parents ought to favour their own children over others' for as long as no standard of minimal decency is breached. Even if we ought to care about everyone, we do not have to care equally.

Let's call the position just described a "partialist" position. Plenty of people provide versions of partialism. Aristotle seems to provide a partialist account of moral obligation, suggesting that wrongs are aggravated by the degree of intimacy between parties: "it is more serious to defraud a comrade than a fellow-citizen, and to refuse help to a brother than to a stranger, and to strike your father than anybody else" (Aristotle, 1976, 1160a1). Presumably, the converse of this is that, whatever our duties to strangers, we have a stronger duty to help a someone close to us, and the closer the association between people, the more they ought to care about whatever rights they have. (That Aristotle cannot be thought of as a believer in free-standing moral duties should not bother us here: the lesson about partiality stands.) David Hume (1711–1776) argues in the same direction, albeit without the normative element, in his *Enquiry*: "sympathy with persons remote from us [is] much fainter than that with persons near and contiguous" (Hume, 1994, p 64). Good Samaritans are admirable largely because their actions exceed those demanded by duty— adequate Samaritans might do no wrong by passing by on the other side if the person in need was not a Samaritan as well.

So I might well be able to come up with a pretty tolerable defence of moral partiality. Transferred to a case such as the provision of healthcare, if we can get the partiality arguments to work, and to work in the right way, we would not have to worry so much about defending the NHS from *prima facie* transnationalism. But they will not work, because exactly what partiality means is still not clear.

Let's start with fairly low ambitions, and say that it is permissible and proper to care more about close friends and family than about strangers. This being the case, we might owe them more than we owe strangers. Making this kind of appeal won't rescue the NHS, though, simply because no account would yet be forthcoming of the moral need for a *national* health service. Appeals to this kind of narrow partiality present a defence for only a *parochial* health service.

Scaling up slightly, we might think that appeals to "the community" would be appropriate, and that we ought to care more about members of our community than about non-members. Taking this on board *would* mean that we were less parochial — but not by all that much. The reason for this is that "community" is an ambiguous word. Strictly speaking, it implies some sort of sharing — to be a member of a community is to have something in common with others; I am in a community with anyone with whom I share some characteristic or with whom I identify in some way. Thus it makes sense to talk about my belonging to the philosophical community; most of my friends and family would not belong in this community, although I could obviously say that we are all members of some other community. At other times, we might talk about humanity, which seems to imply a human community — a group of creatures that has its species or moral status in common. I might belong to several communities, some of which are more morally hefty than others — for example, we might think that, although philosophers might have certain interests, the philosophical community is less morally important than humanity.

But if we understand by "community" something like "those people with whom I identify myself", then whatever the strength of the moral ties between me and my community, they almost certainly will not commit me to the kinds of relationships presupposed by a national health service as it is currently manifested, for the *community* and the *nation* are totally different animals.

For one thing, I do not even know even the name of the people who live a few doors away from me. So we can be described as belonging to the same community only in the most minimal sense that we have some coincident interests (although this applies to pretty much everyone else, too). By contrast, when I travel, I frequently end up chatting to, and exchanging email addresses with, people I meet, and I stay in contact with some of these people after I get home. I might well identify quite closely with these people. In some sense, there is therefore be a strong case for thinking that my foreign friends and I are members of a community in a way that my compatriot neighbours and I aren't. Thus, if one may or ought to care more about members of one's own community than about non-members, and if acknowledging membership of a community has something to do with some kind of identification with people, I might well think that I ought to care more about foreigners whom I know than about neighbours whom, to all intents and purposes, I don't; and, if one of the ways that I manifest my concern about members of my community is to make provision for their access to healthcare, then I might have to make provision for them. But the moral justification for a *national* health service seems not to have got moving. Some compatriots will be the object of my concern, but others — and, in the modern state, this means the vast majority — won't. Some foreigners, too, will be the object of my concern, and, although there probably will be few foreigners in most people's communities, the important point is that nationhood counts for nothing if "community" is supposed to carry the moral burden.

On the other hand, if I identify with other humans, and think of myself as a member of the human community, then this means that there is even less of a moral motor provided for the NHS, since "the nation" would be irrelevant: simply to recognise someone as human would amount to the recognition that we have certain duties to them, among which we might count the provision of at least a certain minimal right to healthcare. I would be committed to all humanity — not just to that small part of humanity that carries a UK passport. *Mutatis mutandis*, the same considerations would come into play if I thought that my need for or right to healthcare was something I held in common with others and that I was a member of something along the lines of a "healthcare recipient" community. Whatever contributions I can be expected to make towards the welfare of members of my community, or with whatever degree of concern I am supposed to regard their rights, to limit myself to the nation lacks coherence.

More colloquially, "community" means "that collection of people with whom we share a social space". In this picture, my community stretches to friends, family, colleagues and neighbours. I do not have to identify particularly *closely* with all the members of my community in this sense. But it should be clear that this understanding of the word "community" will not do that much to provide a moral bulwark for a public health body organised on national lines either. Although identifying a person's community as that group with whom he shares a social space means that we can include many people with whom a person does not identify — and maybe does not know — as a member of his community, and exclude humanity as a whole, this is not enough to warrant a *national* health service. For, once again, a person might well share a social space but not a nationality with someone; and there are still many people with whom he shares a nationality but no social space. So there is still no warrant forthcoming for a national health service.

(Naturally, it would be hopelessly impractical to come up with a reliable way of meeting our obligations to members of the community if the nation has nothing to do with it, so the role for the state in administering welfare at, perhaps, a national level is undiminished. But this is a practical argument about management, not a moral argument in favour of the nation being the primary unit in respect of healthcare provision. The fact that welfare might be managed on a nation-by-nation basis does not indicate that it is defensible for nations to remain aloof of a non-national welfare system, any more than the autonomy of a supermarket manager to run his store as he sees fit warrants a belief that he is not working for a larger organisation that has the capacity to determine what the resources are that he can manage.)

There is one get-out clause here, which is to point out that some people identify closely — or claim to identify closely — with people of the same nationality *just because of* their nationality. A person might point out that, *qua* citizen of the UK, he identifies strongly with other citizens of the UK, and acknowledges his and their membership of a community, *just because* of their common citizenship. If this is the claim, he might be able to say that having nationality in common gives us the right kind of moral tie. However, this sort of person would, in all likelihood, simply be trading on an error.

Not the least of the motivations for this claim is that I think that any such person would have misunderstood the relationship between moral community and nationality: it seems to me that to be a member of a political group such as a nation is to be a member of a kind of community but that one can be a member of a community without being a member of a nation (for an elaboration of which point, see Brassington, 2002). If I am right about this, appeals to the kind of community based on compatriotism would still come up against a more basic question of which communities are the more important: is it my nationality, my profession, my circle of friends or my species that captures the most important of the communities to which I belong? Even allowing the relationship between communities and nations, nationality might simply be one way to understand and unpack "community", and not the most obvious way at that. Thus someone who cares equally about his unknown and his known compatriots or who cares about unknown compatriots more than about known foreigners, and who feels that his moral ties are tighter to those unknown compatriots is, I think, a pretty queer fish.

(Incidentally, this kind of argument should be translatable and applicable to the idea, expressed in the last chapter, that a national health service can be provided with a sure moral footing based on an appeal to civil rights. For civil rights need not have a particular moral justification—they can be simple characteristics of the way a jurisdiction operates. For us to say that a civil right to healthcare is morally important, we would have to be able to give an account of why healthcare is morally important *per se*, so that this importance would filter through to the civil right. But if healthcare is morally important, and granted the foregoing argument about how moral concerns are indifferent to political limits, then it will be important irrespectively of a person's citizenship. In other words, we might have a civil right to healthcare—but this is morally important only insofar as healthcare is morally important independently of political concerns. Absent such non-civil importance, a civil right to healthcare might be politically important, required and admirable —but it is not founded in any positive account of morality and so not amenable to a moral defence.)

The situation in which we find ourselves at the moment is this: if we allow that we have a duty to provide for the welfare of others, there would be a strong reason for there to be a public health service. However, the scope of the service for which we would thereby be arguing either goes a long way beyond a *national* health service, or comes nowhere near it. The closest thing to a moral argument for a national health service rests on the claim that a public health service arranged on national lines might be the best available way for us to discharge our duties given the logistical difficulties in anything else; but, even so, this does not provide all that much of a *moral* argument for a national health service.

The Duties of the State

A shift of emphasis suggests a way in which we might meet a more successful defence of a national health service that is based on an appeal to duties: instead of looking at the duties that individuals have to one another, it might simply be the case that polities have duties towards their citizens, among which is the provision of at least a minimal health service. Such a claim would accommodate the fairly intuitive idea that a government that has the ability to provide welfare for its worst off but that, for some reason, refuses to make such a provision is open to moral criticism; but it would not be as potentially onerous as the outcome of the account that I have been developing up to now. (This is not to say that any polity has to have a particularly *strong* commitment to providing healthcare — it is just that a minimally decent state ought to be prepared to meet the welfare demands of its very worst off, those who need emergency treatment but lack sufficient funds to pay for it, and so on.)

Naturally, it could possibly still be admirable if polities found the resources to contribute to the welfare of non-citizens — but it would not be morally demanded in any way, and things might turn out the other way, too: we might have a reason to withhold our admiration for a polity that donates resources to non-citizens. So we might be able to limit the scope of the provision to within national boundaries. For one thing, a state apparatus the activities of which are motivated by a concern for the welfare of non-citizens might be liable to the charge that it was neglecting its citizens. After all, the demands on any health service tend to be destined to be greater than can practically be met: no matter how much we spend on a health service, there will always be a way for us to spend more. Acting to provide for the welfare of non-citizens, though, suggests that a state is dissipating resources abroad that it could be using to solve domestic problems. For another, given that a polity's provision of basic health care would have to be, at root, publicly funded, it might be that that polity has a duty to minimise the burden on its citizens represented not only by ill health, but also tax. A government that spends money on the welfare of foreigners after having provided a minimal but adequate health system might be thereby wronging its citizens — those to whom its primary duties are addressed — simply by virtue of costing them more than it might. If either of these arguments is sound, while the state might have a duty to provide a health service to its citizens — to all intents and purposes, a national health service — it would have, at most, no duty to provide for the welfare of anyone else, and quite possibly it would have a duty *not* to.

(Some polities might be able to fund their welfare obligations without asking too much in the way of tax: for example, a country might have high oil revenues and a small population. In these cases, though, roughly the same concerns can be put to work. If we think of the oil as a national asset, using the revenue that it generates to fund foreigners' welfare would be either supererogatory or indicative of the government, in whose stewardship the oil is, failing to act in the best interests of those to whose best interests it ought to devote itself;

either way, there is no great moral reason to act in a manner motivated by transnationalism, and possibly a reason to eschew it.)

Would such an account present a serious challenge to the
transnationalist position I have adopted? Probably not. Proponents
of the account would have to answer questions about the provenance of the moral duties of the state. Potentially, we might adopt a
"top-down" model, a "bottom-up" model, or a hybrid. None of
them, though, will provide much of a defence for the nation being all
that morally important.

A top-down model would look like this: the relationship of the
state to the people within it is somewhat analogous to the relationship of a parent to his or her children. In such a system, it would fall
to whoever held power to determine the tone of policy and the
manner in which the state comports itself. But just because the
relationship of state to citizenry is analogous to that of parent to children, it does not follow that the state has duties to its own citizens
and no others, any more than it follows from the fact that a parents
have duties to their own children that they have none to anyone else
or anyone else's children. Of course, the duties that a parent owes to
his or her own children might well dwarf those owed to anyone else.
But the important point is that it is up to a parent to strike a balance,
and there are requirements of minimal decency that obtain in respect
of all children.

If we imagine a situation in which a mother is forced to decide
whether her own child or someone else's is killed by the crazed gun-
man, we would expect her to be most concerned about her own
child: if she was indifferent about which survived, we would think it
improper. But this does not mean that she would have no duties
whatsoever towards anyone else. Given the opportunity to save
both her own child and another person, we would probably think
that she ought not to pass it up. The choice that the mother would
have to make would not be so much one of whose child to save
— there is not much of a choice here — but one of what to do once her
duty to her own child is discharged. And, of course, some duties that
a parent might owe to her child would be nullified in this kind of
situation: playing with one's child might be a duty in some circumstances, but if the mother, having rescued her child, began to play
with it rather than save someone else, we might think that her
priorities were skewed.

So although some of the demands that one child might make on a
mother could properly outweigh those made by another, and

although a mother might have duties to her own child that she does not have to others', other children would not drop out of moral consideration entirely, and there would still be rights and duties that relate to them, such as a duty to ease distress where possible. There would still be a balance to be struck. The same applies in respect of healthcare provision, though. In a top-down state, we might expect the executive to recognise duties to the citizenry and, perhaps, to discharge some of those duties as a matter of priority. But we would also expect non-citizens to have *some* place in moral consideration, and the decision here would be, accordingly, how much of a moral pull is exerted by non-citizens. Though this pull might be less than the citizens', we cannot simply assume that it is negligible unless, *per impossibile*, the executive, monarch, or whoever it is that holds power, has a personal relationship with each and every citizen or subject and none at all — to the extent of being unaware of anything more then the bare theoretical existence of — with any non-citizens or non-subjects.

In a bottom-up state, we would be dealing with a situation in which the state is something that emerges out of a general agreement of people not hitherto living under any jurisdiction: the state would be the product of a social contract. By and large, such states are hypothetical — probably no state has ever been founded in such a way, although social contract thinking played some part in the development of American independence. Clearly, though, the duties of a bottom-up state, even if it is only hypothetical, would represent and reflect the duties of the proto-citizenry in this case.

Whatever duties we would attribute to the state would derive from the original contractors determining that their prospective state would have such duties. Thus, for example, they might decide that one of the things that they want from the state would be healthcare provision for those for whom they care. But, at the same time, the original contractors would have to ask themselves whether their state was meant to serve as a mechanism that could help them more easily discharge their moral duties — perhaps including a duty to provide for others' welfare — or as something that could generate moral duties of its own.

In the former case, there would clearly be no reason to suppose that the duty to provide healthcare could be restricted to the citizenry. After all, the foundation of the state would have been a response to moral duties that one owed to others who, as a matter of definition could not possibly be fellow-citizens, there being no state yet of which anyone could claim citizenship. If the state is something that a group establishes in order better to be able to discharge its moral duties, citizenship turns out really not to be all that important.

In the latter case — if the state is something that generates duties of its own — we are clearly moving back towards the top-down model, in which case we could admit that the state owed its duties primarily to its citizens, but deny that this would mean that it had none to non-citizens. A similar point could be raised if the original contractors decided that the state they were establishing would be such as to provide healthcare to citizens: even if we think that citizenship automatically makes a person more deserving of the state's attention than non-citizens, to decide that the state has no duties at all to non-citizens appears to be arbitrary and therefore indefensible.

Even in a hybrid model of the state, things would not be so different. A hybrid state would be one in which the political balance of power transfers over time to the citizenry from a smaller elite, or to a small elite from the mass of the populace. So, for example, we might imagine a situation in which the citizens of an already-established state decide that the state has an obligation to provide healthcare for them and demand that it does so. In this case, the situation would resemble the top-down model to the extent that the duties in question are those that an already-established state owes to its populace; it would resemble the bottom-up model inasmuch as the moral motor is the populace itself. But none of this would dislodge the idea that, if a state does have a duty to its citizens, it does not have a duty to its citizens *alone*; nor does it dislodge the idea that if citizens can enforce a duty to provide healthcare, it does not follow that they can defensibly restrict its provision to themselves. One cannot simply determine the scope of moral duty by fiat.

The Duty to Transnationalise Health

If we concede that the argument for the public provision of at least a minimal health system can be sustained by means of an appeal to duty, we will find that we have not been arguing for a national health service after all. At is simplest, a duty of beneficence does not imply that there is a significant moral difference between people, and so whatever beneficence we owe to Smith we owe also to Jones, and it does not really matter who Smith or Jones are. This presents a strong *prima facie* case for taking no account of national boundaries in our philanthropy; we would end up with a health service, for sure — but not a *national* health service.

A slightly more sophisticated account of duties of beneficence would be able to make sense of the idea that there is no moral reason to treat everyone in the same way, and that there might even be a moral reason to treat some people differently from others. But, even with this sophisticated argument, the assumption that the scope of a morally-required health service would have a scope even roughly congruent with national boundaries would seem to be unfounded. Whatever the moral weight of compatriotism, it is not sufficient to nullify the moral gravity of people with whom we share membership of some other sort of community, nor to bolster the moral gravity of those with whom we are not.

For the consequentialist, claims about duty might be an elegant fiction, but there is still scope to argue for a "quasi-duty" to provide for the welfare of others based on an appeal to simple optimificity. But the state of the world is such that impartial optimificity seems to be much better served by concentrating on the people in the most need rather than on those with a common citizenship; hence our nascent public health service will have to be transnational in scope; moving away from this to something more nationally based will require moving away from consequentialism. It is this kind of argument that I shall exploit in the next chapter.

Chapter 4

Public Health and Rescue

So far, it would seem that we could appeal to self-interest, to rights, or to duties if we wanted to argue in favour of a publicly-funded health service. What such appeals would not generate, though, would be an argument for a *national* health service. In fact, they would likely be antagonistic to a nationally-focussed system.

The logic that lies behind a national health service must be that the range of people who give us a reason to act, who have a right that is bankable against each of us, or to whom we owe duties, must extend just as much to people that we don't know as to those that we do. Denying that would force us to repudiate a national service in favour of smaller, local health cooperatives. But once we have duties and responsibilities to unknown people, there has to be a limit to these relationships that is congruent with political borders to give us a *national* health service: we have to be able to sustain the claim that unknown compatriots are, in some sense, more important that unknown foreigners. Again, a failure to go along with this undermines the justification for restricting our nascent health service to the nation.

But there is, at the very least, a degree of difficulty in the claim, and there is nothing especially problematic about rejecting it. For it is difficult to see how there is much of a moral difference to be seen between Smith (whom we don't know) and Jones (whom we also don't know but who happens to be a compatriot). Still — let us brush the difficulty to one side and pretend that a person would be *correct* to think that he has an obligation to contribute towards the healthcare of his compatriots that he does not have to foreigners. Noone, I assume, would say that a person has no obligations *at all* towards foreigners — but I shall allow that they are much less weighty than obligations towards compatriots. A question that one

might ask in this case concerns *how much* weightier those duties that
we owe to compatriots are. Presumably there must be some kind of
commensurability between the weight of the duty that we might
owe to one person and that which we might owe to another — for if
there is not, the claim that there is a *difference* in moral weight would
be rendered incomprehensible. If we can say something meaningful
about how much more important compatriots are than foreigners,
though, we could say how much more the British government is
warranted in spending on British needs than on foreign needs,
because we would be able to say, in effect, that one unit of British
suffering is *this* much more demanding than one unit of overseas
suffering, rather as we might say that although every body in space
exerts *some* gravitational pull on us, the Earth's gravitational pull is,
from where we are standing, *this much* stronger than Twearth's.
(Naturally, we could do the same maths in respect of German spending on German needs, and so on for every other country.)

Time, then, for some more figures. Remember that, if you are a UK
citizen, you could have expected in 2003 to have the benefit of annual
health spending worth $2428. The vast majority of this — 85.7% —
was publicly funded, which means that the British benefited from
public healthcare spending worth about $2081 each in that year. At
the same time, the UK government has said that it is aiming to give
foreign aid worth 0.7% of GNI, and a back-of-the-envelope calcula-
tion shows that this represents an aid budget worth a little more than
$212 per capita. (We should not forget that 0.7% of GNI is a *target*
contribution, not a measure of how much actually *is* given: the actual
figure is lower.) So it is clear that UK public spending on health in
2003 amounted to about 9.8 times as much as its aspirational spending on foreign aid.

So, then: allowing that there is a duty of some sort to make foreign
aid available and that aid is only necessary because of a need on the
part of its recipients, and pretending for the sake of the argument
that all foreign aid actually does contribute in a fairly direct way to
the wellbeing of the people receiving it, for the disparity between the
amount that we spend on our own health and welfare and the
amount that we contribute to the health and welfare of the rest of the
world to be defensible, we would have to be able to say that the duty
that UK citizens owe to other UK citizens to provide for healthcare is
a shade under ten times as pressing as is the duty owed to foreigners.

But there is something specious about asking whether the duty
owed to compatriots is 9.8 times more pressing than that owed to

foreigners. For it is clear to most people that, in some parts of the world, people are in a great deal of need, that people in the UK are not in nearly so much need, and that figures and quantifications are as unnecessary as they are ludicrous. We have already seen that the average annual *income* in sub-Saharan Africa in 2003 was about $601, that the average expenditure on health there is about $36, and that, if healthcare could be bought by the kilo, the average UK citizen would buy almost 21 times more of it than the average sub-Saharan African. Life expectancy at birth in 2004 in sub-Saharan Africa was 46 years, as compared to 79 years in the UK, with a mortality rate among the under-5s approaching 30 times the UK figure. Doctors are much scarcer in sub-Saharan Africa (1 per 10 000 people) than in the UK (22 per 10 000). Throwing money at Africa will not solve its problems, but it still does not take much to work out that these figures could be improved with a little more spending either on direct healthcare or on, say, making clean water, sanitation and basic health education more widely available. (Only 58% of sub-Saharan Africans have access to an improved water source, and 36% have access to improved sanitation. The World Bank does not even give figures for the UK.)

Drowning Children and the Duty to Rescue

What impact ought these figures to have on our behaviour? Peter Singer and Peter Unger have both argued that it might very well be wrong for us not to give a lot more away than we do to aid those who are in serious need (Singer, 1972 and 1996; Unger, 1996), and their point translates here. Their arguments hinge on the idea that if we can save a life by making a comparatively small sacrifice, then we ought to do so.

Much of the power of the argument comes from a simple thought experiment: if there is a child drowning in the pond, and we can save that child, we would have to have a very good reason indeed not to do so. We will usually lack any such reason for inaction; letting the child drown is therefore usually inexcusable. The lesson that is drawn from the experiment by Singer and by Unger is that, if not making a comparatively small sacrifice for the sake of saving a life in this instance is inexcusable, we ought also to be prepared to make a sacrifice for the sake of saving other lives. In practice, this means that we ought to be willing to make a sacrifice of some of our wealth for the sake of, say, famine relief in Africa; not to do so would be the equivalent of ignoring the drowning child. The fact that the lives that we save are distant makes no difference, either: Unger's carefully-crafted thought experiments should make that clear. Besides, the fact that we *know* about the needy means that they *are* our moral, even if not our geographical, neighbours.

The relevance of the example to considerations about health spending should be clear. Famine is a pressing concern, but it is also the case that there is a large number of deaths from other causes among the world's poorest that are easily preventable. If deaths from famine (or drowning in ponds) represent a matter of moral concern for us, then so ought any number of other easily preventable deaths; and the simple fact is that large numbers of people die young (and painfully) from diseases that are easily preventable or curable. As a bare statement of fact, this ought to worry any minimally decent person and ought to influence our action, too: specifically, we ought to be prepared to make at least some sacrifice in order to provide a means to rescue people from unnecessary death.

In a sense, this conclusion might appear to be little more than a recapitulation of the argument in the last chapter for there being a duty to contribute to others' welfare. However, the drowning child scenario is more effective, I think, at prompting us to ask *what kind* of contribution to others' welfare we might be expected to make. After all, a duty of beneficence might be discharged by making a contribution to charity or paying into a national (or transnational) insurance scheme; but it might also be discharged by *campaigning* for more welfare provision. But to mount a water-safety campaign when faced with a drowning child would clearly be an inappropriate response: something much more direct is needed. Acting out of a concern for others' welfare often means that we have to be prepared to make a sacrifice—but not all sacrifices are alike. Just as campaigning for water safety when faced with drowning child would represent our making a sacrifice, but the *wrong* one, so there are certain sacrifices in relation to real suffering that would be misdirected.

Healthcare Spending and Rescue

What kind of sacrifice might we be expected to make? Singer's suggestion is that, all else being equal, a contribution equivalent to 10% of our income to the world's neediest would satisfy the demands of minimal decency (Singer, 1996, p 246), but that many of us ought to be willing to sacrifice a good deal more; almost certainly, we ought to be more circumspect about whether we really do need that new car, the overseas holiday, the sophisticated stereo and so on. We may dispute the figures and insist that there is nothing wrong with having more of a concern for our own welfare than for others' without having to worry about doing damage to the gist of the argument. Spending more on ourselves and those we love than on those whom we have never met is not incompatible with spending more on those whom we have never met all the same, perhaps thereby foregoing the opportunity for something good for ourselves or those we love. In the overwhelming number of cases, our lives would not really suffer.

If we are convinced by the argument from rescue, we might find ourselves in a position in which we can argue for something like the philanthrotax that I considered in chapter 3, with the proviso that the money raised thereby would be ringfenced to provide either basic healthcare or the means to improve health (such as improved sanitation) for the world's needy. As with the philanthrotax system, there need be no particular barrier to the supposition that people could opt out; but there need be no reason either to suppose that it is all that important for them not to have any option but to pay it, on the assumption that virtuous people would pay the extra anyway and that autonomy need not be infringed by a limit on the number of alternatives from which a person can choose. Some people might think that it is important that we be allowed to act as we please, whether our actions be virtuous or vicious. But consequentialists at least are also likely to admit that there could be situations in which the importance of unfettered action is dwarfed by the importance of optimific action. Alternatively, if the idea of extra taxation is not attractive, we could still argue for what amounts to the same thing: that a slightly lower proportion of an unchanged tax bill be spent on public institutions — including bodies such as the NHS — and the difference spent overseas. The difference would be little more than a small sacrifice from our pay cheques, or a slightly smaller range of treatments available from the local clinic.

We ought to bear in mind here that, in contributing to the NHS, we are already making a sacrifice for the sake of others' welfare. The rescue argument simply raises the question of whether the funds raised are all that well distributed. Importantly, if people have a right to basic healthcare, or if we have a duty to provide basic healthcare, then we are *more* than meeting our obligations to some people through our spending on bodies like the NHS, which could permissibly be much more basic than the body that exists today: for example, what orthodontic work is carried out on the NHS is unlikely to count as a basic requirement—people can and do lead tolerably good lives even with badly-aligned teeth—and the same might go for, say, the removal of a cataract from a person whose other eye still has good vision. Of course, it is a good thing if we can provide orthodontic work to everyone and cataract operations to everyone; and it is admirable that we do so. But there will be a good number of cases in which making such provision is supererogatory.

At the same time as we are more-than-meeting some of our obligations, we are arguably not meeting our obligations to some others. The World Health Organisation estimates that 1.16 million African newborns die every year, but that 800 000 of these deaths could be prevented if established interventions were made more widely available (WHO, 2006, pp 5, 9, 18, 20, 152)—and, of course, we may assume that the health of those who would have survived anyway would still be improved. Widening the provision of basic but essential maternal, newborn and child health packages to cover 90% of mothers and babies in Africa would come at a cost, admittedly: about $1 billion. But a sense of perspective is required here: that $1 billion amounts to $1.39 per recipient, and counts as cheap in comparison to the roughly $150 billion (that is, $2428 each for a population of around 60 million) that the UK spends each year on its own healthcare. Even if the bill were to be footed by the UK alone, it would work out at costing UK citizens less than $17 each (that is: less than 1% of the amount that we already contribute to the NHS). Once again, if we find the drowning child scenario compelling, we ought seriously to suppose that not to make this kind of payment towards saving or significantly improving Africans' lives problematic. We probably ought to think that the differential between our health spending on ourselves and on foreigners is in need of rebalancing and that, to the extent that it is ill-balanced, it is indefensible.

The Meteorite Argument

Another way to frame the argument would be based on imagining that a meteor has fallen on a part of the town where you live, causing significant damage. In response to the disaster, the council offers the electorate a choice: either it can introduce a large increase in its tax burden in order to pay for repair work, or else it can approve a plan that would see things like the promised new playgrounds and overhaul of the kitchens in council houses shelved, thereby freeing up resources for repair work. After all, important as playgrounds and kitchens are, something more pressing has cropped up. Either way, sacrifices must be made. We would probably say that anyone who tried to raise a serious complaint about the diversion of funds had failed to see some part of the moral picture. Had people been injured in the disaster, we might feel similarly that healthcare resources could — and ought — to be diverted. Orthodontic work and cataract operations might become less of a priority if the resources that we intended to devote to them suddenly became needed for emergency relief of some kind — especially if that relief promised to prevent a good number of deaths. After all, we presumably think it good — or, at least, acceptable — to contribute to provide for orthodontic work or cataract operations because we think that others' welfare is important; but if we think that others' welfare is important, there would seem to be no reason at all for the welfare of the meteorite's victims across town not to figure in our considerations. Probably, we would think the plight of the meteorite's victims poorer than that of those with crooked teeth.

But there is a disaster the effects of which we could mitigate by diverting funds from those treatments at home that are admirable but to which people arguably have no inalienable or overriding right: it is difficult to see how the levels of poverty and disease in Africa and other parts of the world are anything but a disaster. And even if foreigners — for the sake of the argument — properly exert less of a moral pull on us than do compatriots, what is important is that they still do exert *some* kind of moral pull. So the question that we must ask is whether the moral gravity of foreigners is so diminished by their distance as to mean that the failing sight and poor teeth of our compatriots is the more pressing concern. Given that most people think that death is not only worse, but *much* worse than losing the sight in one eye or having misaligned teeth, there seems little doubt that, frequently, we ought at least to consider spending less money on non-essential treatments on the NHS to which there is little compelling right, and diverting the funds that we would have spent on these treatments to life-saving treatments or the provision of the means to prevent natural deaths in, say, sub-Saharan Africa. The alternative is that each of us should be prepared to make an additional sacrifice, which, for the sake of ease, could be administered by way of a philanthrotax.

Put another way, if we are willing to make a sacrifice for the sake of non-essential treatments, we ought not to object to our sacrifice being used instead for essential ones: we might well find that there is something morally odd about our willingness to contribute to the

NHS' ability to provide non-life-saving procedures when we contribute so little to life-saving interventions overseas. Caring more
about ourselves than about strangers is fine, but it doesn't warrant
ignoring those strangers' needs entirely, and a public health service
that discounts foreigners' welfare just because they are foreign
would appear to exclude them from the public in a manner that is not
only arbitrary, but also incoherent—for how can one be expelled
from the public?

Similar considerations apply in respect of other forms of treatment, which we may find that we ought at least to consider foregoing in order to save the lives of some of the world's poorest. For
example, a course of IVF costs around £3000, and has about a 28%
success rate; under current guidelines (I am writing in 2006), all
women with appropriate clinical need should have at least 1 cycle of
treatment paid for by the NHS. The rationale must be that such
spending is justified. But is it? Without a doubt, having a child is
enormously important to many people, and the inability to conceive
may be a source of distress. Moreover, it is also true that, in many
cases, having a child is something that improves the lives of its
parents enormously. But, still, there is a question to be asked about
whether the £3000 per course might be better spent elsewhere—
perhaps overseas. There is good reason to suppose that it might,
especially given the plausible claim that, if we were to choose not to
pay for IVF but to spend the money overseas, we would not be
depriving anyone of a right (much less of a child) that they might
otherwise reasonably expect to have had; we would not make them
worse off. We would simply not be compensating for a piece of bad
luck.

Granted, by not providing Africans with clean water, we would
also not be depriving them of anything that they would otherwise
have had. But this is something of a red herring; for, if we had the
resources, there might be a better argument for providing IVF to all
who need it—or even only *really want* it. What counts, though, is that
resources are limited, and so, granted that we want to maximise
welfare, the relevant question is who would be benefited the most
from our spending. It is unlikely to be the infertile couple, however
unfortunate and distressing their situation.

With this in mind, I think that I can make my position a bit tougher
to defend and suggest that there could even be some are *life-threatening* conditions that we ought perhaps to forego treating when doing
so will free funds to spend overseas. Some forms of cancer are more

serious than others: many men die *with* prostate cancer, for example, but such is the nature of the disease that comparatively few die *from* it: it simply develops too slowly in the majority of cases to present an immediate threat. Nevertheless, a diagnosis of the condition often leads to surgery. But why? A programme of active surveillance would mean a patient submitting to a blood test every few months, and perhaps a biopsy every couple of years to ensure that the cancer had not become more active; if it had not, no treatment would be offered. Certainly, this would mean many men not receiving cancer treatment, and it would therefore compel him to live with a life-threatening condition. But it would be a lot cheaper, freeing up funds to save lives that *are* in danger. (And, incidentally, the men in question might be better off, since prostate surgery brings with it the risk of bladder problems and impotence: if the cancer was not an immediate threat, we might well feel that it is better not to have to face these risks.)

Maybe this position is still too easy to defend — after all, prostate cancer is often not immediately life-threatening, and, as the picture stands, it would still be removed were it to become so. Finally, then, what about refusing to treat some conditions that *are* more straight-forwardly life-threatening — say a prostate cancer that has started to become more vigorous, or another kind of cancer? Would it be deeply wrong to refuse to treat a life-threatening cancer so that the money can be spent overseas? Perhaps sometimes. But even allow-ing (for the sake of the argument) that foreigners exert less moral gravity than compatriots, there are considerations that force us at least to ask searching questions about who should benefit from our money, such as the number of lives that could be saved by spending, say, £1000. Will it be more in the UK or Africa, and what is the "dis-count rate" for foreigners? We might also want to consider the likeli-hood of that money achieving what we want it to: writing in *New Scientist* in March 2006, and citing studies in *The Lancet*, Ralph Moss questions the effectiveness of Herceptin, the breast cancer drug that a number of women have gone to court to have provided on the NHS; providing improved water and sanitation, by contrast, is of proven effectiveness. Another consideration might be the age of the people saved. Providing clean water can save a child from dying of diarrhoea; adults tend not to be so vulnerable to this. By contrast, things like cancer, stroke and so on are more of a threat to us as we age. But there is a strong intuition that a child's death is worse than an adult's (this is sometimes articulated as a "fair innings" argument);

so even if £1000 spent anywhere and on anyone was just as likely to save the same number of lives, we might still think that we ought to spend it on the young because the number of extra years lived would thereby be maximised.

These questions are difficult and concern emotive issues. But it would be facile to suppose that difficulty and emotion might provide us with reasons not to face a problem. Certainly consequentialism forces us to ask these questions; and asking them simply reflects the considerations about optimificity that I mentioned in the last chapter. If we are concerned about making the world as good a place as possible, we cannot help but to consider the possibility that we would wring much more good from each unit of health spending in sub-Saharan Africa than we would from the same amount of spending in western Europe.

I am not claiming here that we definitely ought not to provide cancer treatment and orthodontic work on the NHS. Rather, there is more of a rhetorical challenge being offered: how can we justify not spending a small amount each to save many lives in Africa given that we are prepared to make a sacrifice to provide for a range of treatments in the UK that are, arguably, inessential, unreliable, or not enormously cost-effective? Is there any defence for keeping the balance of our spending as it is? Or might it be the case that, while there is a moral argument for a public health service—or even a national one—the manner in which it gobbles up public health resources is unjustifiable?

Objections

There is likely to be a couple of objections levelled here. In the first, the thought might be that people *do* have a right to infertility treatment, cancer treatment and so on, and that this has to weigh importantly: so importantly that we cannot simply demand that they sacrifice their right—and potentially their life. This may be a civil right or a human right. But, either way, my response to this claim is simply to deny it. It does not follow from accepting that people have a right to healthcare that we must accept that they have a right to all kinds of healthcare. Rights-claims, as a rule, are at their most secure when they are at their most minimal. I have to admit that I have difficulty seeing how one might have a right to all possible healthcare interventions.

But even if there *is* a right to all possible healthcare interventions, then it can surely only be a *prima facie* right, rebuttable in certain situations — the meteorite argument should have demonstrated this. When healthcare resources are scarce — as they are — and when making resources less scarce has to be balanced against another *prima facie* right — in this case, the right not to be forced to make *too* much of a sacrifice — it will simply be impossible to satisfy all rights claims. And since *ought* is usually taken to imply *can*, it would follow that we are under an obligation to satisfy only those claims that we reasonably can, given other obligations that we might have.

Moreover, noone is required to sacrifice his life, even if a significant slice of the health budget ends up being spent overseas: what is sacrificed is, at most, the opportunity to have his life saved. Why does this sacrifice not fall on the Africans whose lives we *are* trying to save, though? Simply because — as I claimed a moment ago — the argument from rescue is directed at securing the best possible outcome from an imperfect initial situation; on this basis, it seems reasonable to assume that we ought to do whatever produces the best outcome. If a better outcome is achieved by spending money on healthcare in the UK, then that is where it should be spent. If Africa, then Africa. The chances are it will be Africa.

By analogy, if we are able equally easily to save one person whom we know and like or one stranger from drowning, we might opt to save our friend; we might even have an obligation to act in this way. But when the choice is between *possibly* saving our friend and *almost certainly* saving a boatload of strangers, and if we find the argument from rescue compelling, I think that we might have to have a very good reason indeed still to try to save our friend. And if it's a stranger or a boatload of strangers, it would be perverse to choose the one over the many. How, then, are we to justify failing to make a sacrifice to provide reliable interventions to many people when we are willing to make a sacrifice to provide less reliable interventions for fewer, as is the case when we pay (comparatively) so much for the NHS aid and so little towards foreign aid?

The other objection is that, in having contributed to national insurance schemes and the like, British people have an entitlement to getting a commensurate return from the NHS; meanwhile, not having paid national insurance, foreigners have no such entitlement.

This objection fails in a number of ways, though. In the first place, we might wonder whether the money that we pay into the health system, though often spoken of in terms of national insurance, really is any such thing; or whether it is a means of buying entitlement; or whether it is, in fact, simply a necessary part of the discharge of the duties that we have to each other *qua* constituent members of the public sector. If the last of these descriptions is accurate, the fact that we have paid into the system will *not* generate an entitlement — all it will do is discharge a duty — and entitlement, in turn, will have nothing to do with having paid. (By analogy, discharging our duty to rescue the child from the pond will not mean that we are entitled to demand anything of her or her guardians in return — not even gratitude.)

If the second of the descriptions is accurate, and national insurance payments are simply a means of building up an entitlement, then there certainly would be little or no scope to send the funds raised overseas. But, by the same token, there would be no scope for anyone to say that he was entitled to any treatment that cost more than he had contributed (or could reasonably be expected to contribute). Hence the illest might well find that they could not rely on healthcare being available, and those whose lifestyle was such as to minimise their risk of needing significant medical help might well feel that they had the right to make a lower contribution than those with an unhealthy lifestyle or congenital health problem. In other words, if building up an entitlement or being expected to repay the public sector for treatments we received, say, as a child is an important consideration, we would expect to see a very different kind of NHS.

Finally, if contributions are properly understood as insurance, this might debar foreigners from benefiting and would (probably) allow for the congenitally ill or constitutionally vulnerable to claim healthcare that they might not otherwise be able to afford. In this version of affairs, some people would still suffer from the misfortune of having been born in a part of the world where such insurance was not available, or beyond their reach. But this looks like a world in which people can be, in effect, medically disenfranchised as a result of actions or inactions in which they played no relevant part; maybe this is something that we will have to accept. But more ought to be said here.

Since contributions to the NHS are compulsory, we are clearly dealing in this picture with a compulsory insurance scheme. But the notion of compulsory insurance is odd: given a presumption that people ought to be able to spend their money as they wish, there is a puzzle about why health insurance should be treated any differently. Maybe (we might say), at least minimal health insurance ought to be compulsory because, if a person were to be hit by a bus, it would be incumbent upon us to provide for him at least emergency treatment, for which we ought to be able to recoup the cost. This line of argument is initially attractive. But it does not militate against the idea that, should someone be in need, we have a duty to rescue them that is irreducible to their entitlement. For as long as it is the case that it would be obscene for an ambulance driver or doctor to check someone's wallet to make sure that he had the relevant insurance cover before administering life saving treatment, it must also be true that ability to pay is not the primary concern here. Moreover, it would be no less obscene for a doctor to abandon the uninsured person who needs life-saving treatment in favour of the person with insurance whose treatment is only life-enhancing. There is a chance that the effort will go unrewarded—but that, in the end, is not an excuse for failing to provide what most people would rightly think constitutive of minimal decency.

On all accounts—whether we go for the first, second or third interpretation, we cannot help but to arrive at the idea that the NHS is indefensibly inconsistent in its position: the argument from rescue forces some serious questions to be asked about the prioritisation of health spending, and hints that a body such as the NHS cannot defend spending so much on one group of people—the population of the UK—and so little on another— the sick and starving of Africa— if it is really there as a public service directed at providing welfare. It would still seem incumbent on the global public sector (of which the NHS represents a part) to accept the sacrifices necessary to fund improved, but still only basic, healthcare provision around the world. In other words, even if the *principle* of an NHS does, after all, have a decent moral basis—perhaps drawing from some kind of argument about civil rights to healthcare—the way it works out practically may still present us with moral problems.

Summary

Where Does This Leave Us?

Throughout this book, I have not really been trying to argue that it is *wrong* for us to distribute our spending as we do. Rather, I have been asking whether, if we accept proposition *A*, there is any defence for not accepting proposition *B* as well, even though *B* might be unexpected (and maybe even unwelcome). I have been suggesting that, by and large, whatever rationale might be offered for the formation of a public health service such as the NHS, there is at least an equally good one to think that attaching the word "national" to a public health service lacks robust moral backing.

In chapter 1 I claimed that, if the rationale behind the formation of a publicly-funded health service is self-interest, it would be irrational of us to think of this service as nationally based. Depending on the extent and nature of our contact with the outside world, we ought rather to have our eye on a service that is either more parochial than a national service would be, or on one that has a much wider reach. The health service that it would be rational to promote would be related to national concerns only insofar as it might well fall to national governments to administer a service that would be, at heart, non-national.

An appeal to rights as the foundation of a national health service has more going for it on the face of things. Certainly, an appeal to healthcare as a human right generates an argument for a public health service that is free at the point of access. What it does not do, though, it tell us that this service should be organised nationally: an appeal to human rights is an appeal to something that takes no account of political borders. Thus to limit the scope of the health system that might be founded on an appeal to human rights to a *national* health system seems to lack justification. Again, there might be practical reasons to give states authority over how they run the public health system as it would appear in their jurisdiction—but this does not generate a *moral* reason to keep things nationally based; it is compatible with these practical concerns to suppose that the role of the state would simply be an administrative part of a larger project to provide healthcare—perhaps a country's health budget could be based on contributions to a transnational agency, or at least distributed *as if* that were the case.

In chapter 2, I had quite a lot to say on the theme of human rights. However, one thing that I did not look at in particular depth was the supposition that healthcare might be something that we can claim courtesy of civil, rather than human, rights—although if we agree (as I suspect most would) that there would be something blameable about a government that chose to stop making healthcare provision, we are probably making an implicit appeal to non-civil rights.

Still, if healthcare is a civil right, then an appeal along these lines would be much better at generating an argument for a national health service. But this would not be the whole story; for, in chapter 4, I suggested that there may be circumstances in which a person's rights, whether civil or non-civil, can be overridden by other concerns such as would mean that, although the *idea* of a national health service could stand, we would have to ask serious questions about how it is run. On this suggestion, there might be nothing problematic with the notion of a health service run on national lines, but there might be a problem with investing so much in ourselves and so little in others. The *idea* of the NHS would remain intact, but the practical application of that idea would be indefensible.

Meanwhile, we might deny that there is any right to healthcare at all. This would not mean that there is no argument for a public health service, for such a body might be demanded by an account of the duties that we owe each other. If there is a duty to provide for others' welfare, though, it is unlikely that this would be limited (or stretched) to national borders. If an account of duties provides the moral motor for our action, there is not likely to be a defence available for a *national* health service. Such was the argument of chapter 3.

The conclusion is, then, that the NHS as it stands lacks all that good a moral defence. I have no wish to say that there should not be an NHS—but, all the same, there are conceptual problems with drawing too close an association between moral concerns and political concerns; and solving these problems by adverting to the idea that healthcare is a civil right does not avoid worries about the moral permissibility of a health service that provides as much as it does to some people while many others are left to die needlessly even if they have no bankable right to be saved. The NHS represents a partial response to the moral demands that we face; but those same demands generate a reason to look transnationally.

What is to be Done?

One might think that I am making the suggestion that, on the basis of the foregoing argument, we should be forced to suspend spending on the NHS until sub-Saharan Africa has the same number of GPs and functioning MRI scanners as the rest of the world. Perhaps an argument could be made for governments being morally obliged to contribute the revenues they collect for healthcare purposes to a central pool where they could be redistributed according to need. I am making no such suggestion: such an argument would be unwieldy and probably unsuccessful, especially given my sympathy for partialism in chapter 3. (There are also quite tenable arguments against egalitarianism that may be invoked.)

Moreover, I am willing to suspend my idealism and relinquish any claim that we should spend even as much on aid to the rest of the world *in toto* as we do on the NHS. Still, vaccination programmes are cheap; water filters are cheap; mosquito nets are cheap; education is cheap: we might not have to in order to make a significant difference. According to the UN, meeting Millennium Development goals for safe water and sanitation by 2015 would cost around $11.3 billion per year — this sounds a lot, but we ought to bear in mind for the sake of comparison that the UK public sector spends about $120 billion per year on the NHS already, supplemented by extra private healthcare spending — and the estimated return on the money spent on water and sanitation would be $84 billion. Spread throughout the OECD, the sacrifice of providing water would be noticeable, but probably not unbearable.

For sure, the OECD would not be the main recipient of benefit — but I do not benefit particularly from my national insurance contributions paying for insulin for diabetics I have never met, and so if it is acceptable for a national health service to shunt funds around like this, then it is presumably also acceptable for a transnational body to shunt them around as well. Money spent on basic healthcare overseas would make far more of a difference than the same amount spent on whizz-bang medical equipment here — 1.1 billion people lack clean water, and about half of the world's hospital beds are filled by people suffering from water-borne diseases. The practical problems about spending the money are real — but there is no reason why we can't treat the UN as the executive arm of the global public (just as we treat the UK government as the executive arm of the UK public) and the WHO as a Transnational Health Service in waiting once the money is there.

Presumably, the government and the UN both think that 0.7% of GNI represents a decent level of donation for the developed world to make in foreign aid and all that is morally required, since that is the stated aspirational level of donation. But by cutting per capita spending on the NHS by 10% and transferring it to overseas aid, we could give away 1.4% of GNI — double the minimum necessary — and we would still have almost $1800 to spend on ourselves. If we think that Singer's argument is powerful — and, remember that he suggests that we ought to be prepared to give away 10% of our wealth, so 1.4% of GNI might not be all that onerous — we ought to think that not doing this, and keeping the NHS budget as it is, would be indefensible. That doesn't mean that it's *wrong*, of course: it simply means that the moral argument has not been fully developed.

(A similar point about budget-balancing could, of course, also be used in respect of, say, defence spending — except that noone pretends that defence spending is directly aimed at welfare provision. Health spending clearly is, and so we are already committed to the idea that welfare spending is a good thing if we think that the public sector ought to pay something towards health in a way that we are not when we talk about defence.)

We should be clear that the question that I am asking is not whether or not someone ought to receive treatment: it is whether or not someone ought to receive *this particular* treatment, given a range of other details concerning the world in which we find ourselves. When we are talking about an expensive treatment for cancer, or about procedures that can counter low levels of fertility, it would be, fairly uncontroversially, a good thing if they could be made available to everyone who wanted them and for whom they were suitable. But it is worth repeating a point that I made in the introduction to this book. There, I suggested that it might well be unreasonable to deny to an 80-year-old the magic potion that would give him five extra years of life if there was no competition for it. Where there is competition for it, and depending on the nature of the competition, the reasonable thing might be to give the potion to someone else, or even not to buy it at all.

If we had the resources to ensure that to everyone in the world had access to a reasonably long life of reasonable quality, public spending on expensive cancer treatments would be a lot more reasonable. A reasonably long life does not have to be as long as that enjoyed by people in the most developed parts of the world, either; nor does a reasonable quality of life have to be of the same quality of life enjoyed by the most privileged. However, it would probably be longer and of a higher quality than that which is lived by a good number of people in the poorest parts of the world today. Therefore it seems that, until most people do experience improvements in the length and quality of their lives, there is a lot to be said for the idea that, while spending on the NHS is all very well, its importance is trumped by other things. Spending quite as much as we do on healthcare in the UK, and as little as we do on healthcare overseas, is indefensible.

Further Reading

Almond, B (1993) "Rights" in Singer, P (ed.) *A Companion to Ethics* (Malden, MA: Blackwell)

Aristotle (1976) *Ethics* (Harmondsworth: Penguin)

Aristotle (1992) *The Politics* (Harmondsworth: Penguin)

Brassington, I (2002) "Global Village, Global *Polis*" in Norman, R and Moseley, A (eds.), *Human Rights and Military Intervention* (Aldershot: Ashgate)

Brassington, I (2006) "Globalisation and the Moral Indefensibility of the NHS" (unpublished, but available via http://www.brighton.ac.uk/cappe/presentations/Brassington_Globalisation_and_the_Moral_Indef ensibility_of_the_NHS.pdf)

Frankfurt, H (1969) "Alternate Possibilities and Moral Responsibility", *Journal of Philosophy*, vol. 66, # 23

Hobbes, T (1996) *Leviathan* (Cambridge: Cambridge UP)

Hume, D (1994) *Enquiry Concerning the Principles of Morals* (La Salle: Open Court)

Kant, I (1993) *Grounding for the Metaphysics of Morals* (Indianapolis: Hackett) [1]

Kant, I (1996) *The Metaphysics of Morals* (Cambridge: Cambridge UP)

Locke, J (1960) *The True End of Civil Government* in Barker, E (ed.) *Social Contract* (London: Oxford UP)

Mill, JS (1998) *Utilitarianism* in Mill, JS *On Liberty and Other Essays* (Oxford: Oxford World's Classics)

Moss, R (2006) "Hype and Herceptin", *New Scientist*, vol. 189, # 2541

Nozick, R (1974) *Anarchy, State and Utopia* (New York: Basic Books)

Paine, T (1985) *Rights of Man* (Harmondsworth: Penguin)

Rawls, J (1999) *A Theory of Justice* (Oxford: Oxford UP)

Singer, P (1972) "Famine, Affluence and Morality", *Philosophy and Public Affairs*, vol. 1, #1

[1]   Note that, throughout the text, I have given references to Kant in the form *x:y* rather than as conventional page numbering. This represents the standard Prussian Academy pagination which can be found printed down the margins of most editions of Kant's work, and which is therefore more useful for tracking down references across different translations and editions. The same applies to my citations of Aristotle, which adopt, as far as possible, the Bekker system of referencing as reproduced in most translations.

Singer, P (1996) *Practical Ethics* (Cambridge: Cambridge UP)

Unger, P (1996) *Living High & Letting Die: Our Illusion of Innocence* (New York: Oxford UP)

Wilkinson, S (1999) "Smokers' Rights to Health Care: Why the 'Restoration Argument' is a Moralising Wolf in a Liberal Sheep's Clothing", *Journal of Applied Philosophy*, vol. 16, #3

World Bank (2006) *World Development Indicators 2006* (Washington DC: World Bank)

World Health Organisation (2006) *Opportunities for Africa's Newborns* (Geneva: World Health Organisation)

Much of the "raw" information I used in this book is available online: listed below are the most valuable sites that I used.

CBI data about days lost to illness are available via
http://www.cbi.org.uk/ndbs/press.nsf/0363c1f07c6ca12a8025671c003 81cc7/1fba36cf7478790180257168004aab8a?OpenDocument

The NHS' claim about healthcare as a human right can be found on its website:
http://www.nhs.co.uk/England/AboutTheNhs/CorePrinciples.cmsx #a

The Universal Declaration of Human Rights is available from many sources; among these is: http://www.un.org/Overview/rights.html

The development data that I have used can be found in various places on the World Bank's website; useful starting points are:
http://devdata.worldbank.org/hnpstats/cd.asp
http://web.worldbank.org/WBSITE/EXTERNAL/DATASTATISTICS /0,,contentMDK:20415471~menuPK:1390200~pagePK:64133150~piPK: 64133175~theSitePK:239419,00.html
http://devdata.worldbank.org/hnpstats/HNPSummary/countryData /GetShowData.asp?sCtry=GBR,United%20Kingdom

UN data concerning the availability of water and the consequences of its lack are summarised at
http://www.un.org/waterforlifedecade/factsheet.html

Information about the cost of IVF came from the website of the Human Fertilisation and Embryology Authority:
http://www.hfea.gov.uk/cps/rde/xchg/SID-3F57D79B-8C03902A/hf ea/hs.xsl/406.html

The WHO's *Opportunities for Africa's Newborns* is downloadable as a pdf via
http://www.who.int/pmnch/media/publications/africanewborns/e n/index.html

Index

SOCIETAS: essays in political and cultural criticism

Public debate has been impoverished by two competing trends
On the one hand the trivialization of the media means that in-depth commentary has given way to the ten second soundbite. On the other hand the explosion of knowledge has increased specialization, and academic discourse is no longer comprehensible.

This was not always so — especially for political debate. But in recent years the tradition of the political pamphlet has declined. However the introduction of the digital press makes it possible to re-create a more exciting age of publishing. *Societas* authors are all experts in their own field, but the essays are for a general audience. The books are available retail at the price of £8.95/\$17.90 each, or on bi-monthly subscription for only £5/\$10. Details at **imprint-academic.com/societas**

IMPRINT ACADEMIC, PO Box 200, Exeter, EX5 5YX, UK
Tel: (0)1392 851550   Fax: (0)1392 851178   sandra@imprint.co.uk